HISTORY OF PSYCHOPHARMACOLOGY

VOLUME 4

Index

HISTORY OF PSYCHOPHARMACOLOGY

VOLUME 4

Index

Spanish Edition Editors:
Francisco López-Muñoz
Cecilio Álamo

English Edition Editor:
Edward F. Domino

NPP Books
http://www.nppbooks.com

Original version in Spanish. Historia de la Psicofarmacología, 3 tomos, directores F. López Muñoz and C. Álamo González. Copyright © 2007 Editorial Médica Panamericana S.A., ISBN 84-7903-458-0. Av. Alberto Alcocer 24, 28036 Madrid, Spain

NPP Books, 15 Sunset Road, Arlington, MA 02474, USA, www.nppbooks.com

Ordering Information:
For individual sales, this book is available for sale through www.nppbooks.com, or writing to the publisher at the address above. For quantity sales, special discounts are available on quantity purchases by corporations, associations, and others. For details, contact the publisher at the address above. For orders by U.S. trade bookstores and wholesalers. Please contact: Lightning Source Inc. (US), 1246 Heil Quaker Blvd, La Vergne, TN USA 37086, Email: inquiry@lightningsource.com

Printed in the United States of America, and the United Kingdom.

Publisher's data

History of Psychopharmacology.
F. López Muñoz, C. Álamo González, E.F. Domino, editors.

International Standard Book Numbers:

Volume	Hardcover	Softcover
Set of all volumes	978-0-916182-29-8	978-0-916182-30-4
1	978-0-916182-21-2	978-0-916182-25-0
2	978-0-916182-22-9	978-0-916182-26-7
3	978-0-916182-23-6	978-0-916182-27-4
4	978-0-916182-24-3	978-0-916182-28-1

Library of Congress Control Number: 2013940078

1. History. 2. Medical.

Acknowledgements

The publishers of the Spanish version are greatly acknowledged for permitting this English version of their superb original three volumes.

A total of four volumes cover the subject matter. Each chapter represents the efforts of the authors who wrote the original drafts. Any errors are the responsibility of the Editor and should be communicated to the Editor and contact author of each respective chapter.

The Spanish to English translation of each chapter was first done by Michelle Hunscher. Subsequently many individuals modified various chapters to make the text easier for an average layperson to read and understand the complex mechanisms by which drugs act in the brain. The efforts by Carmen Allen, Terry L. E. Butcher, Candra Gill, Priya Goel, Neetu Gulati, Lynne May, Adrian Miller, Cassandra Miller, and Jessica Walsh produced the initial draft of the book in English. Subsequently, Lisa Chen, Kenneth E. Domino, and Zarina G. Memon, as Copy Editors, made numerous corrections that resulted in the current revision. In the process, the nuances and feelings of the Spanish language may have been replaced by less expressive English text. The unique design of the volume covers was motivated by Figure 1–1, which depicts Pinel freeing the insane from their chains. Ken Domino and Zarina Memon took as many figures from the book and created the mosaic shown on the front, spine, and back cover of each volume. Use a hand lens to discover the many images that depict over the centuries the people and drugs involved in psychopharmacology. Volume 4 contains an index of the first three volumes, created by Ken Domino.

Dedication

These four volumes are dedicated to the students and staff, academic and nonacademic, past, present, and future, of a remarkable history of the development of psychoactive drugs. Each chapter is written by experts in the field who have documented their knowledge. A special thanks to each of them, and Prof. F. López-Muñoz and C. Álamo González Editors of the Spanish original works.

* * * *

Editor – E. F. Domino, M.D.

Contents of Volume IV

Contributors

Francisco José de Abajo Iglesias
Department of Pharmacology, Faculty of Medicine, University of Alcalá, Alcalá de Henares, Madrid, Spain

Cecilio Álamo González
Department of Pharmacology, Faculty of Medicine, University of Alcalá, Alcalá de Henares, Madrid, Spain

Simona Albu
Brief Therapy Reception Center (CATEB), Esquirol Hospital, Saint-Maurice, France

Rafael Aleixandre Benavent
Institute of the History of Science and Documentation, University of Valencia-CSIC, Valencia, Spain

Luis F. Alguacil Merino
Department of Pharmacology, Pharmaceutical Technology and Development, Experimental Sciences and Health Faculty, San Pablo CEU University, Boadilla del Monte, Madrid, Spain

Doug Andrews
North Coast Area Health Service, Rural Clinical School, University of New South Wales, Coffs Harbour, Australia

Ramón Antequera Recio
Forensic Medicine Institute of Ciudad Real and Toledo Justice State Office, Ciudad Real, Spain

Juan José Arechederra Aranzadi
Psychiatry Service, Ramón y Cajal, University Hospital, Madrid, Spain

Spilios V. Argyropoulos
Home Treatment Team, South London and Maudsley Hospital, NHS, Croydon, United Kingdom

Francisco Arias Horcajadas
Psychiatry Service, Alcorcón Hospital Foundation, Alcorcón, Madrid, Spain

Belén Arranz Martí
Parc Sanitari Sant Joan de Déu, CIBERSAM, Barcelona, Spain

Hans-Jörg Assion
LWL-Klinik, Dortmund, Germany

Sofia Avissar
Department of Pharmacology, Ben, Gurion University of the Negev, Beer Sheva, Israel

Thomas A. Ban
Vanderbilt University, Nashville, Tennessee, United States

Josep Lluís Barona Vilar
Institute of the History of Science and Documentation, University of Valencia-CSIC, Valencia, Spain

Alan A. Baumeister
Department of Psychology, Louisiana State University, Baton Rouge, Louisiana, United States

Per Bech
Psychiatric Research Unit, Frederiksborg General Hospital, Hillerød, Denmark

Joseph Benyaya
Department of Neuroscience, Janssen-Cilag, Issy-les-Moulineaux, France

Miquel Bernardo Arroyo
Psychiatry Service, Institute of Psychiatry and Psychology, Hospital Clinic, Barcelona, Spain

German E. Berrios
Department of Psychiatry, University of Cambridge, Addenbrooke's Hospital, Cambridge, United Kingdom

Vinod S. Bhatara
Department of Psychiatry, University of South Dakota, Sioux Falls, United States

Carlos Bocos de Prada
Department of Biology, Faculty of Pharmacy, San Pablo CEU University, Boadilla del Monte, Madrid, Spain

Jesús Boya Vegue
Department of Cell Biology, Faculty of Medicine, Complutense University, Madrid, Spain

Paolo Brambilla
Department of Pathology and Medicine, Clinical and Experimental (DPMSC), Section of Psychiatry, University of Udine, Udine, Italy

Frank P. Bymaster
Department of Psychiatry, Faculty of Medicine, Indiana University School of Medicine, Indianapolis, United States

José Cabrera Forneiro
National Institute of Toxicology, Madrid, Spain

Joseph R. Calabrese
Department of Psychiatry, School of Medicine, Case Western Reserve University, University Hospitals of Cleveland, Cleveland, United States

Helena M. Calil
Department of Psychobiology, Paulista School of Medicine, Federal University of Sao Paulo, Sao Paulo, Brazil

Ricardo Campos Marin
Center for Human and Social Sciences, Higher Council for Scientific Research (CSIC), Madrid, Spain

Liliana M. Cancela
Department of Pharmacology, Faculty of Chemical Sciences, National University of Cordoba, Argentina

Elisaldo A. Carlini
Department of Psychobiology, Paulista School of Medicine, Federal University of Sao Paulo, Sao Paulo, Brazil

Eva Ceskova
Department of Psychiatry, Faculty of Medicine, Masarykova University, Brno-Bohunice, Czech Republic

Georges Chapouthier
Centre Emotion, CNRS USR 3246, Pavillon Clerambault, Hôpital Salpêtrière, Paris, France

Lara Chayab
Department of Pharmacology, University of Toronto, Toronto, Canada Neuropsychopharmacology Research Program, Sunnybrook and Women's College Health Science Centre, Toronto, Canada

Patrick Clervoy
Department of Psychiatry, Saint-Anne Hospital, Toulon, France

Jean M.H. Conemans
Department of Pharmacy and Toxicology, Hospital Pharmacy Noordoost-Brabant, Hertogenbosch, The Netherlands

Olga Cuenca Cot
J.A. Llorente & Cuenca, Communication Consultants, Madrid, Spain

Eduardo Cuenca Fernández
Department of Pharmacology, Faculty of Medicine, University of Alcalá, Alcalá de Henares, Madrid, Spain

Antonio Diéguez Gómez
Department of the History of Science, Institute of History, Higher Council for Scientific Research (CSIC), Madrid, Spain

Rebeca Díez-Alarcia
Department of Pharmacology, University of the Basque Country (UPV/EHU), Leioa, Bizkaia, Spain

Edward F. Domino
Department of Pharmacology, University of Michigan, Ann Arbor, United States

Michael Dudley
Department of Psychiatry, Prince of Wales Hospital, School of Psychiatry, University of New South Wales, Sydney, Australia

Nady el-Guebaly
Department of Psychiatry, University of Calgary, Alberta Health Services-Foothills Medical Centre, Calgary, Canada

Eric A. Engleman
Department of Psychiatry, Faculty of Medicine, Indiana University School of Medicine, Institute of Psychiatric Research, Indianapolis, Indiana, United States

Peter Fangmann
LWL-Klinik Bochum, Department of Psychiatry, Psychotherapy, Psychosomatic and Preventive Medicine, Ruhr University, Bochum, Germany

Miguel Fernández Braña
Department of Chemistry, Experimental Sciences and Health Faculty, San Pablo CEU University, Madrid, Spain

Jennifer L. Francis
Department Medical and Clinical Psychology, Uniformed Services University of the Health Sciences, Bethesda, United States

Filiberto Fuentenebro de Diego
Department of Psychiatry and Psychology, Complutense University, Madrid, Spain

Federico Gago Bádenas
Department of Pharmacology, University of Alcalá, Alcalá de Henares, Madrid, Spain

Margarita García-Amador
Psychiatry Service, Gregorio Marañón General Hospital, Madrid, Spain

Pilar García-García
Department of Pharmacology, University of Alcalá, Alcalá de Henares, Madrid, Spain

Francisco García-Valdecasas[1]
Department of Pharmacology, University of Barcelona, Spain

José Manuel Goikolea Alberdi
Biomedical Research Institute Agusti Pi I Sunyer (IDIBAPS), Bipolar Disorders Program, Hospital Clinic, University of Barcelona, Spain

Moran Golan
Department of Clinical Biochemistry and Pharmacology, Faculty for Health Sciences, Ben-Gurion University of the Negev, Israel

Ángel González de Pablo
History of Science, Epidemiology and Public Health, Unit of History of Science, Faculty of Medicine, Complutense University, Madrid, Spain

Julio González Iglesias
Department of the History of Dentistry, Alfonso X El Sabio University, Villanueva de la Cañada, Madrid, Spain

Carmen González-Martín
Department of Pharmacology, Pharmaceutical Technology and Development, Experimental Sciences and Health Faculty, San Pablo CEU University, Boadilla del Monte, Madrid, Spain

Eduardo González Martínez
Judicial Police Group of Guardia Civil, Castilla - La Mancha Criminology Scientific Association, Valdepeñas, Ciudad Real, Spain

Marina Gordaliza Escobar
Department of Pharmaceutical Chemistry, Pharmacy Faculty, University of Salamanca, Spain

Ali Gorji
Institute of Physiology, University of Münster, Germany

[1]Deceased.

Todd D. Gould
Department of Psychiatry & Pharmacology and Experimental Therapeutics, University of Maryland School of Medicine, Baltimore, United States

Bernard Granger
Department of Psychiatry, Tarnier Hospital (Gpe Hospitalier Cochin), Paris, France

José Antonio Guerra Guirao
Department of Pharmacology, University of Alcalá, Alcalá de Henares, Madrid, Spain

Mike F. Hawkins
Department of Psychology, Louisiana State University, Baton Rouge, United States

Rafael Huertas García-Alejo
Center for Human and Social Sciences, Higher Council for Scientific Research (CSIC), Madrid, Spain

Matti Isohanni
Department of Psychiatry, Faculty of Medicine, University of Oulu, Finland

Akio Itoh
Department of Pharmaceutical Sciences, Faculty of Pharmacy, Meijo University, Japan

Gordon F.S. Johnson
Department of Psychological Medicine, University of Sydney, Australia

Alberto R. de Juan
Department of Physiology, National Technological University, Buenos Aires, Argentina

Peter W. Kalivas
Department of Neuroscience, Medical School, Medical University of South Carolina, Charleston, United States

Kenneth C. Kirkby
Department of Psychiatry, School of Medicine, University of Tasmania, Hobart, Australia

Hwee-Ling Koh
Department of Pharmacy, Faculty of Science, National University of Singapore, Republic of Singapore

Hannu Koponen
Department of Psychiatry, Faculty of Medicine, University Hospital of Kuopio, University of Kuopio, Kuopio, Finland

Mónika Erika Kovács
Institute of Behavioral Sciences, Semmelweis University, Budapest, Hungary

Susan G. Leckband
Department of Veterans Affairs, Health System (VAHCS), San Diego, United States

Anton J.M. Loonen
Halsteren and Department of Pharmacy, University of Groningen, Groningen, The Netherlands

María Inés López-Ibor Alcocer
Department of Psychiatry and Medical Psychology, Faculty of Medicine, Complutense University, Madrid, Spain

Juan José López-Ibor Aliño
Institute of Psychiatry and Mental Health, San Carlos Clinical University Hospital, Department of Psychiatry and Psychology, Faculty of Medicine, Complutense University, Madrid, Spain

Francisco López-Muñoz
Faculty of Health Sciences, Camilo José Cela University, Villanueva de la Cañada, Madrid, Spain
Department of Pharmacology, Faculty of Medicine, University of Alcalá, Madrid, Spain

José Ramón López-Trabada
Addictive Behavior Unit, 12 de Octubre University Hospital, Madrid, Spain

Rodrigo Machado-Vieira
Laboratory of Neuroscience (LIM-27), Department and Institute of Psychiatry, University of Sao Paulo, Sao Paulo, Brazil
Experimental Therapeutics and Pathophysiology Branch, National Institute of Mental Health, Bethesda, United States

Mariano Madurga Sanz
Division of Pharmacoepidemiology and Pharmacovigilance, Spanish Agency for Medicines and Healthcare Products, Majadahonda, Madrid, Spain

Rafael Maldonado López
Department of Experimental and Health Sciences, University Pompeu Fabra, Barcelona, Spain

Gin S. Malhi
CADE Clinic, Department of Academic Psychiatry, Royal North Shore Hospital St Leonards, Discipline of Psychiatry, University of Sydney, Australia

Jacques Mallet
Molecular Genetics Laboratory of the Neurotransmission and Neurodegeneration Processes (LGN), National Center for Scientific Research (CNRS) UMR 7091, Bât CERVI, Pitié-Salpêtrière Hospital, Paris, France

Husseini K. Manji
Johnson & Johnson Pharmaceuticals Group, Titusville, New Jersey, United States

Iris Manor
Geha Mental Health Center, Petach Tikva, Israel, Department of Psychiatry, Sackler Faculty of Medicine, Tel-Aviv University, Tel-Aviv, Israel

Jorge Manzanares Robles
Institute of Neuroscience, Miguel Hernandez University – CSIC, San Juan, Alicante, Spain

Belén Martín-Águeda
Teaching and Research Unit, Castilla – La Mancha Health Service, Guadalajara, Spain

Yolanda Martín Sánchez-Cantalejo
Sciences Department, Polytechnic High School, European University of Madrid, Villaviciosa de Odon, Madrid, Spain

José Martínez-Pérez
Area of the History of Science, Faculty of Medicine of Albacete, University of Castilla - La Mancha, Albacete, Spain

José Javier Meana Martínez
Department of Pharmacology, University of the Basque Country (UPV/EHU), CIBERSAM, Leioa, Bizkaia, Spain

Juan Medrano Albéniz
Gasteiz-Centro Mental Health Center, Alava Mental Health Services, Vitoria, Spain

Jonathan M. Meyer
Department of Psychiatry, University of California, San Diego
VAMC, Psychiatry Service, San Diego, California, United States

Jouko Miettunen
Department of Psychiatry, Faculty of Medicine, University of Oulu, Oulun Yliopisto, Finland

Philip B. Mitchell
School of Psychiatry, University of New South Wales, UNSW School of Psychiatry, Prince of Wales Hospital, Randwick, Australia

Hans-Jürgen Möller
Department of Psychiatry, University of Munich, München, Germany

Dolores Montero Corominas
Division of Pharmacoepidemiology and Pharmacovigilence, Spanish Agency for Medicines and Healthcare Products, Majadahonda, Madrid, Spain

José Manuel Montes Rodríguez
Department of Psychiatry, South-East Hospital, Arganda del Rey, Madrid

Daniel Monti
Mercy Behavioral Health, Pittsburgh, United States

Jaime M. Monti
University of Montevideo, Department of Pharmacology and Therapeutics, Health Clinic, Montevideo, Uruguay

Luis E. Montiel
History of Science, Epidemiology and Public Health, Unit of History of Science, Faculty of Medicine, Complutense University, Madrid, Spain

Lidia Morales Goyanes
Department of Pharmacology, Pharmaceutical Technology and Development, Experimental Sciences and Health Faculty, San Pablo CEU University, Boadilla del Monte, Madrid, Spain

Pedro Moreno Gea
Balearic Institute of Psychiatry and Psychology, Palma de Mallorca, Spain

Carlos A. Morra
Department of Psychiatry, Faculty of Medicine, National University of Cordoba, Instituto Neuropsiquiátrico Privado, Córdoba, Argentina

Sagrario Muñoz Calvo
History of Pharmacy Unit, Department of Public Health and the History of Science, Faculty of Pharmacy, Complutense University, Madrid, Spain

Toshitaka Nabeshima
Department of Regional Pharmaceutical Care & Sciences, Meijo University, Tenpaku-ku, Nagoya, Japan

Tamás Gergely Nagy
Department of Neurology and Psychiatry, Health Services District 13, Budapest, Hungary

Claudio A. Naranjo
Department of Psychiatry and Medicine, University of Toronto
Neuropsychopharmacology Research Program, Sunnybrook Health Sciences Centre, Toronto
Clinical Pharmacology Program, Addiction Research Foundation, Toronto, Canada

Pentti Nieminen
University of Oulu, Medical Informatics and Statistics Research Group, University of Oulu, Finland

Philippe Nuss
Psychiatry Service, Saint Antoine University Hospital Centre (CHU), Saint Antoine, Paris, France

Ahmed Okasha
World Health Organization Collaborating Center for Research and Training in Mental Health,

Okasha Institute of Psychiatry, Ain Shams University, Cairo, Egypt

Óscar Olías Calvo
Psychiatry Service and Research Unit, 12 de Octubre University Hospital, Madrid, Spain

Jesús Pascual Arriazu
Expert Group on Addictive Behaviors (GECA), Madrid, Spain

Carmen Pérez-García
Department of Pharmaceutical Sciences, Faculty of Pharmacy, San Pablo CEU University, Boadilla del Monte, Madrid, Spain

José Ramón Pigem Palmés
Bellavista Psychiatric Clinic, Lleida, Spain

Herman M. van Praag
Department of Psychiatry and Neuropsychology, University Hospital Maastricht, Research Institute Brain and Behavior, Maastricht University, The Netherlands

Beatriz Puente Ballesteros
Department of Sinology, Faculty of Arts, Katholieke Universiteit Leuven, Belgium

Jorge A. Quiroz
Translational Medicine Leader, Pharma Research & Early Development, Neuroscience, Hoffman-La Roche Inc., Nutley, United States

Jean-David Rafizadeh-Kabe
Pharmaceutical Research Institute (PRI), Bristol-Myers Squibb, Wallingford, United States

Dilip Ramchandani
Department of Psychiatry, Drexel University College of Medicine, Merion Station, United States

Alfonso Rodríguez Pascual
Pharmacoepidemiology and Pharmacovigilance Division, Spanish Agency for Medicines and Healthcare Products, Majadahonda, Madrid, Spain

Tushar Roy
Department of Cardiology, National Heart Institute, New Delhi, India

Vandana Roy
Department of Pharmacology, Maulana Azad Medical College, University of Delhi, New Delhi, India

Gabriel Rubio Valladolid
Department of Psychiatry, "Doce de Octubre" University Hospital, Complutense University, Madrid, Spain

Jerónimo Saiz Ruiz
Psychiatry Service, Ramon and Cajal University Hospital, University of Alcalá, Madrid, Spain

Luis San Molina
Department of Child and Adolescent Psychiatry, Hospital Sant Joan de Déu, Esplugues de Llobregat, Barcelona, Spain

Marsal Sanches
UT Center of Excellence on Mood Disorders, Department of Psychiatry and Behavioral Sciences, Medical School, University of Texas, Houston, United States
Department of Psychiatry, Santa Casa de Sao Paulo School of Medicine, Federal University of Sao Paulo, Brazil

David Sanger
Psychiatry Service, Saint Antoine University Hospital Centre (CHU), Saint Antoine, Paris, France

Fernando Santander Cartagena
Alava Mental Health Services, Vitoria, Spain

Gabriel Schreiber
Department of Psychiatry, Health Sciences Faculty, Ben-Gurion University of the Negev, Beer Sheba, Israel
Barzilai Medical Center, Ashkelon, Israel

Winston W. Shen
Department of Psychiatry, Wan Fang Hospital, Taipei Medical University, Taipei, Taiwan

Jair C. Soares
UT Center of Excellence on Mood Disorders, Department of Psychiatry and Behavioral Sciences, Medical School, University of Texas, Houston, United States

Theodore L. Sourkes
Department of Psychiatry, McGill University, Montreal, Canada

Dan J. Stein
Department of Psychiatry and Mental Health, Groote Schuur Hospital, University of Cape Town, South Africa Mt. Sinai Medical School, New York, United States

Konstantin V. Sudakov
Anokhin Institute of Normal Physiology, Russian Academy of Medical Sciences, Moscow, Russia

Steven T. Szabo
Psychiatry and Behavioral Sciences, Duke University Medical Center, Durham, North Carolina, United States

Chay-Hoon Tan
Department of Pharmacology, Yong Loo Lin School of Medicine, National University of Singapore, Republic of Singapore

Tilli Tansey
History of Modern Medical Sciences, School of History, Queen Mary, University of London, London, United Kingdom

Shigenobu Toda
Department of Psychiatry and Neurobiology, Kanazawa University School of Medicine, Ishikawa, Japan

Siegfried Tuinier[2]
Vincent van Gogh Institute for Psychiatry, Centre of Excellence for Neuropsychiatry, Venray, The Netherlands

Samuel Tyano
Geha Mental Health Center, Petah Tikva, Israel
Department of Psychiatry, Sackler Faculty of Medicine, Tel-Aviv University, Tel-Aviv, Israel

---

[2]Deceased.

Ronaldo Ucha-Udabe[3]
Member of the World Health Organization in Psychopharmacology and Biological Psychiatry, National University of Buenos Aires, Argentina Ex-Chairman of the History Committee for the Collegium Internationale Neuro-Psychopharmacologicum (CINP), Nashville, United States

Donald R.A. Uges
Department of Pharmacy, Toxicology, and Forensic Medicine, University Medical Center Groningen, University of Groningen, The Netherlands

Leyre Urigüen Echeverría
Department of Pharmacology, University of the Basque Country - Euskal Herriko Unibertsitatea, Leioa, Spain

Juan Carlos Valderrama Zurián
Institute of the History of Science and Documentation, University of Valencia – CSIC, Valencia, Spain

Julio Vallejo Ruiloba
Psychiatry Department, University Hospital of Bellvitge, L'Hospitalet de Llobregat, University of Barcelona, Spain
President of the Spanish Society of Psychiatry

Alfonso Vázquez Moure
Comprehensive Care Center for Drug Addicts (CAID), Alcalá de Henares, Madrid, Spain

Alfonso Velasco Martín
Department of Cell Biology, Histology, and Pharmacology, Faculty of Medicine, University of Valladolid, Spain

Patrice Venault
Centre Emotion, CNRS USR 3246, Pavillon Clerambault, Hôpital Salpêtrière, Paris, France

Willem M.A. Verhoeven
Vincent van Gogh Institute for Psychiatry / Erasmus University Medical Centre, Centre of Excellence for Neuropsychiatry / Department of Psychiatry, Venray, The Netherlands

Eduard Vieta Pascual
Biomedical Research Institute Agusti Pi i Sunyer (IDIBAPS), Bipolar Disorders Program, Hospital Clinic, University of Barcelona, Spain

Lucinda Villaescusa Castillo
Department of Pharmacology, University of Alcalá, Alcalá de Henares, Madrid, Spain

[3] Deceased.

Randall Webber
Lighthouse Institute, Chestnut Health Systems, Bloomington, Illinois, United States

William L. White
Senior Research Consultant, Chestnut Health Systems, Port Charlotte, Florida, United States

David T. Wong
Department of Psychiatry, Faculty of Medicine, Indiana University School of Medicine, Indianapolis, Indiana, United States

Ana Isabel Wu-Chou
Department of Psychiatry, Taipei Medical University-Wan Fang Medical Center, Taipei, Taiwan

Wai-Ping Yau
Department of Pharmacy, Faculty of Science, National University of Singapore, Republic of Singapore

Francisco Zaragozá García
Department of Pharmacology, Faculty of Medicine, University of Alcalá, Alcalá de Henares, Madrid, Spain

Carlos A. Zarate, Jr.
Experimental Therapeutics & Pathophysiology Branch, Division Intramural Research Programs, National Institute of Mental Health, Bethesda, Maryland, United States

Contents of All Volumes

VOLUME I

THE ORIGINS OF SCIENTIFIC MEDICINE:
BIOLOGICAL PILLARS ON THE BIRTH OF
PSYCHOPHARMACOLOGY

SECTION I

History of Psychiatry

1. Brief History of Psychiatry
   *Antonio Diéguez, Ricardo Campos,
   Rafael Huertas*

SECTION II

**"Psychoactive" Substances before the
Development of Psychoactive Drugs: The
Origins of Scientific Medicine**

2. Treatment of Mental Illness in Ancient
   and Medieval Times
   Ángel González de Pablo

3. Psychopharmacology during the Renaissance
   *Luis Montiel, Beatriz Puente-Balles-
   teros*

4. Responses to Deviant Behavior: The
   Use of Drugs in the Treatment of In-
   sanity in the Nineteenth Century
   José Martínez-Pérez

5. Psychopharmaceuticals in the Nineteenth and Early Twentieth Centuries
   Sagrario Muñoz

SECTION III

**Basic Research and its Contribution to
the Advance of Psychopharmacology**

6. The Contribution of the Neuro-
   sciences to the Evolution of Psy-
   chopharmacology
   *Luis F. Alguacil, Carmen Pérez-García,
   Lidia Morales, Carmen González-
   Martín*

7. Neuron Theory: Antecedents, Postu-
   lates and Historical Relevance
   Jesús Boya, Francisco López-Muñoz

8. Theory of Functional Systems: A New Contribution to Neuroscience and Psychopharmacology
   Konstantin V. Sudakov

9. Advances in Neurochemistry: The Mechanism of Action of Psychotropic Drugs as a Neurotransmitter-Receptor Interaction
   José Javier Meana, Rebeca Diez-Alarcia

10. Intracellular Neurobiology as a Future Challenge for Psychopharmacology
    Jorge A. Quiroz, Rodrigo Machado-Vieira, Steve T. Szabo, Todd D. Gould, Carlos A. Zarate, Husseini K. Manji

11. From the Discovery of DNA to the Genomic Era: Psychopharmacology "á la carte"
    Jacques Mallet

12. The Legacy of Pharmaceutical Chemistry in Psychopharmacology
    Miguel F. Braña, Marina Gordaliza, Yolanda Martín

13. A Brief History of Pharmaceutical Analysis Technologies and its Contribution to Psychotropic Drug Discovery and Development
    Hwee-Ling Koh, Wai-Ping Yau, Chay-Hoon Tan

14. The History of Therapeutic Drug Monitoring of Psychotropic Drugs
    Anton J.M. Loonen, Jean M.H. Conemans, Donald R.A. Uges

15. Animal Models of Mental Illness from a Historical Perspective
    Jorge Manzanares, Óscar Olías, Leyre Urigüen

SECTION IV

Contribution of Clinical Disciplines to the Development of Psychopharmacology

16. Clinical Trials with Psychotropic Drugs from a Historical Perspective: Methodological Progress
    Claudio A. Naranjo, Lara Chayab

17. Advances in Statistical Methodology and its Significance in the Development of Psychopharmacology
    Pentti Nieminen, Jouko Miettunen, Hannu Koponen, Matti Isohanni

18. The Role of Imaging Techniques in the Development and Clinical Use of Psychotropic Drugs
    Marsal Sanches, Paolo Brambilla, Jair C. Soares

SECTION V

History of Biological Theories of Mental Disorders

19. Historical Development of the Monoamine Hypothesis of Schizophrenia
    Alan A. Baumeister, Mike F. Hawkins, Jennifer L. Francis

20. Monoamines and Depression: A Retrospective
    Herman M. van Praag

21. GABAergic Neurotransmission and Anxiety Disorders: A Historical Approach
    Patrice Venault, George Chapouthier

22. Etiopathic Hypothesis of Substance Abuse Disorders
    Peter W. Kalivas, Liliana M. Cancela

VOLUME II

THE REVOLUTION OF PSYCHOPHARMA-
COLOGY: THE DISCOVERY AND DEVEL-
OPMENT OF PSYCHOACTIVE DRUGS

SECTION VI

**"The Revolution of Psychopharmacol-
ogy": History of Drug Treatment of
Psychiatric Disorders**

23. Psychopharmacology: The Beginning
    of a New Discipline
    Thomas A. Ban

24. Antipsychotics (I). The Origins of the
    Antipsychotic Era: The Discovery of
    the Neuroleptic Properties of Reser-
    pine
    *Vinod S. Bhatara, Francisco López-
    Muñoz, Cecilio Álamo*

25. Antipsychotics (II). Chlorpromazine
    and the Origin of Antipsychotic Drugs:
    From Antihistamines to Phenoth-
    iazines
    *Patrick Clervoy, Jean-David Rafizadeh-
    Kabe*

26. Antipsychotics (III). The Consolida-
    tion of Neuroleptic Therapeutics: Clin-
    ical Introduction of Haloperidol and
    Butyrophenones, and Development of
    Thioxanthenes
    *Bernard Granger, Simona Albu, Joseph
    Benyaya*

27. Antipsychotics (IV). A History of
    Clozapine and Concepts of Atypicality
    Jonathan M. Meyer

28. Antidepressants (I). From Antituber-
    cular Drugs to Hydrazidic Antidepres-
    sants and Other MAOIs
    Hans-Jürgen Möller

29. Antidepressants (II). Imipramine and
    the Origin of Antidepressant Drugs:
    From Antihistamines to Heterocyclic
    Antidepressants
    Peter Fangmann, Hans-Jörg Assion

30. Antidepressants (III). The Triumph of
    Psychotropic Drugs Rational Design
    Policy: Fluoxetine Discovery and SSRI
    Clinical Introduction
    *Eric A. Engleman, David T. Wong,
    Frank P. Bymaster*

31. Antidepressants (IV). New Mecha-
    nisms of Action and New Families of
    Antidepressant Drugs
    Eva Ceskova

32. Mood Stabilizers (I). Discovering of
    Antimanic Properties of Lithium Salts
    Gordon F.S. Johnson

33. Mood Stabilizers (II). Valproic Acid and
    Carbamazepine as Agents for Bipolar
    Disorder: Historical Perspectives
    *Ana Isabel Wu-Chou, Winston W. Shen,
    Francisco López-Muñoz, Cecilio Álamo*

34. Mood Stabilizers (III). New Anticon-
    vulsants and Antiepileptic Drugs as
    Mood Stabilizers
    *Eduard Vieta, José M. Goikolea, Gin S.
    Malhi, Joseph R. Calabrese*

35. Anxiolytics (I). The Meprobamate Dis-
    covery and the Beginning of the Anxi-
    olytic Era
    Dilip Ramchandani

36. Anxiolytics (II). The Consolidation of the Anxiolytic Era: Development and Clinical Introduction of the Benzodiazepines
Philippe Nuss, David Sanger

37. Anxiolytics (III). Non-Benzodiazepine Anxiolytics: An Uncertain History Not Yet Finished
Spilios V. Argyropoulos

38. Sedatives and Hypnotics (I). The Psychiatric History of Bromides and Chloral Hydrate
Theodore L. Sourkes

39. Sedatives and Hypnotics (II). The Relevant Historical and Pharmacological Role of the Barbiturates
Ronaldo Ucha-Udabe, Francisco López-Muñoz, Cecilio Álamo

40. Sedatives and Hypnotics (III). New Non-Benzodiazepine Hypnotic Agents
Jaime M. Monti, Daniel Monti

41. History of Pharmacological Treatment for Substance Use Disorders
William L. White, Randall Webber

SECTION VII

Other Pharmacological Approaches in Psychiatry

42. Biological Therapies before the Introduction of Modern Psychotropic Drugs
Philip B. Mitchell, Kenneth C. Kirkby

43. Central Nervous System Stimulants
Luis F. Alguacil, Carmen Pérez-García, Lidia Morales

44. History of Anti-Aggression Drugs
Siegfried Tuinier, Willem M.A. Verhoeven

45. Pharmacological Therapy of Cognitive Disorders: A Challenge for Psychopharmacology
Akio Itoh, Toshitaka Nabeshima

46. Endocrine and Immunological Treatments in Psychiatry: Historical Aspects
Tamás G. Nagy, Mónika E. Kovács

47. Opioid Drugs: Past, Present, and Future
Rafael Maldonado, Francisco López-Muñoz

48. The Discovery of Anesthetics and Their Relationship to Psychiatry
Julio González

49. Phytotherapy and Psychiatry
Francisco Zaragozá, Lucinda Villaescusa

SECTION VIII

Drugs and Psychotropic Drugs: A Historical Relationship

50. Drugs as Psychotropic and Neurotoxic Substances: A Brief History of Drug Use
José Cabrera Forneiro

51. Use of Drugs of Abuse in the Treatment of Mental Illness (I). Alcohol and Tobacco as Therapeutic Agents through History
Gabriel Rubio, José Ramón López-Trabada, Jesús Pascual, Francisco López-Muñoz

52. Use of Drugs of Abuse in the Treatment of Mental Illness (II). Opiates, Cannabis, Stimulants and Hallucinogens
José Ramón López-Trabada, Gabriel Rubio, Jesús Pascual, Alfonso Vázquez

53. Psychotomimetic Agents. Discovery and History of LSD-25
Patrick Clervoy, Jean-David Rafizadeh-Kabe

54. Psychoactive Drugs and Their Mechanisms of Dependence: Benzodiazepines, an Existing Debate
Luis San, Belén Arranz

VOLUME III

THE CONSOLIDATION OF PSYCHOPHARMACOLOGY AS A SCIENTIFIC DISCIPLINE: ETHICAL-LEGAL ASPECTS AND FUTURE PROSPECTS

SECTION IX

Public and Private Institutions and the Advancement of Psychopharmacology

55. The Pharmaceutical Industry's Role in the Development of Psychopharmacology
Tilli Tansey

56. The NMDA Antagonists Phencyclidine, Ketamine, and Dizocilpine: Examples of Pharmaceutical Industry/Academic Interaction in the Development of Psychopharmacology
Edward F. Domino

57. The Contribution of Scientific and Professional Associations to Advance Psychopharmacology
Nady el-Guebaly

58. The Role of Health Administration in the Development of Psychopharmacology: Regulatory Aspects and Pharmacovigilance
Francisco J. de Abajo, Mariano Madurga, Alfonso Rodríguez, Dolores Montero

SECTION X

Ethics in Psychopharmacology

59. History of Ethics in Psychopharmacology
Ahmed Okasha

60. Ethics in Psychiatric Research and its Relation to the Psychotropic Drugs: From the Nuremberg Code to the Madrid Declaration
Francisco López-Muñoz, José A. Guerra, Pilar García-García, Belén Martín-Águeda, Cecilio Álamo

61. Ethics in the Prescription of Psychotropic Drugs: Historical Aspects and Current Implications
Cecilio Álamo, Francisco López-Muñoz, Pilar García-García, Eduardo Cuenca

SECTION XI

Law and Psychopharmacology

62. Legal Aspects of Psychopharmaceutical Research: Clinical Tests and Informed Consent from a Historical Perspective
Juan J. Arechederra, Francisco Arias

63. Historical Perspective of the Legal Aspects of Psychopharmacological Treatments: Information, Voluntariness, and Competence
Juan Medrano, Fernando Santander

64. Mind Altering Agents and Criminology: Historic Myth or Reality?
Eduardo González, Francisco López-Muñoz, José A. Guerra, Ramón Antequera

65. The Political and Institutional Abuses of Psychotropic Drugs
Michael Dudley, Doug Andrews

SECTION XII

The Contribution of Psychopharmacology to the Development of Psychiatry

66. Social and Health Consequences of Clinical Introduction of Psychotropic Drugs
Kenneth C. Kirkby

67. Psychopharmacology and the Stigma of Mental Illness
Juan J. López-Ibor, Olga Cuenca, María I. López-Ibor

68. Role of Psychotropic Drugs in Quality of Life Improvement in Psychiatric Patients: Historical Aspects
Per Bech

69. The Contribution of Psychopharmacology to Current Psychiatric Nosology
Jerónimo Saiz, José M. Montes

SECTION XIII

Miscellaneous

70. The History of Electroconvulsive Therapy and Its Nexuses with Psychopharmacology
Margarita García-Amador, Ramón Pigem, Miquel Bernardo

71. The Role of Serendipity in the Ontogenesis of Modern Psychopharmacology
Alan A. Baumeister, Mike F. Hawkins

72. The Placebo in Psychiatry: Historical Perspective
Vandana Roy, Tushar Roy

73. Psychopharmacology and Psychotherapy: The Symbol of Serpents
Samuel Tyano, Iris Manor

74. Evolutionary Theory and Psychopharmacology
Dan J. Stein

75. The History of Psychopharmacology in Non-Occidental Cultures
Ali Gorji

76. The Non-Psychiatric Uses of the Psychotropic Drugs from a Historical Perspective
Cecilio Álamo, Francisco López-Muñoz, Eduardo Cuenca

77. Some Psychotropic Drugs as Poisons: Historical Role and Literary and Cultural Relevance
Alfonso Velasco

SECTION XIV

Present and Future of Psychopharmacology

78. Etiopathogenic Hypothesis of Mental Disorders at Present: The Role of Classical and New Neurotransmission and Neurotransduction Systems
Gabriel Schreiber, Moran Golan, Sofia Avissar

79. The Contribution of Genomic and Proteomic Techniques to the Study of the Pathogenesis of Mental Disorders and to the Development of Psychopharmacology
Luis F. Alguacil, Carmen Pérez-García, Carlos Bocos, Gonzalo Herradón, Shigenobu Toda

80. Novel Computer-Based Technologies in the Rational Design of Psychiatric Drugs
Federico Gago

81. Pharmacology of Cerebral Activity
Francisco García-Valdecasas, Eduardo Cuenca, Cecilio Alamo, Francisco López-Muñoz

82. The Internet and the Information Revolution: Their Relevance to Psychopharmacology
Pedro Moreno

83. New Perspectives in Psychopharmacology
Cecilio Álamo, Francisco López-Muñoz, Eduardo Cuenca

SECTION XV

Psychopharmacology in Spain and Latin

America

84. A Brief History of Spanish Psychiatry: The Historical Origins
Josep L. Barona, Juan C. Valderrama, Rafael Aleixandre

85. The History of Psychopathology in Spain
Juan J. López-Ibor, Filiberto Fuentenebro

86. History of Preclinical Psychopharmacology in Spain
Francisco López-Muñoz, Eduardo Cuenca, Cecilio Álamo

87. Psychopharmacology in Latin American from a Historical Perspective
Ronaldo Ucha-Udabe, Helena M. Calil, Elisaldo A. Carlini, Alberto R. de Juan, Carlos A. Morra

VOLUME IV

INDEX

Index

Symbols

α-ethyltryptamine, 2-538
    etryptamine, 2-12, 2-107
    Monase, 2-538
α-secretase, 2-390
β-CCM, 1-509–1-513
β-amyloid, 2-388–2-391
β-carboline, 1-307, 1-509
    alkaloids, 2-236, 3-797
β-dystrobrevin, 3-509
β-endorphin, 1-222, 1-243, 2-422, 3-645
β-lipotropin, 1-221
β-secretase, 2-389, 2-390
β-site-APP-cleaving enzyme, 2-390
γ-aminobutyric acid (GABA), 1-205,
        1-241, 1-242, 1-268, 1-307,
        1-329, 1-352, 1-422, 1-447,
        1-451, 1-505–1-508, 1-511, 1-
        512, 1-514, 1-531, 2-15, 2-96,
        2-150, 2-206, 2-208–2-210,
        2-235, 2-236, 2-247, 2-249,
        2-293, 2-312, 2-313, 3-505,
        3-521, 3-527, 3-596, 3-598,
        3-600, 3-604, 3-605, 3-610,
        3-660, 3-662–3-664
    receptor
        $GABA_A$, 1-268, 1-269, 1-324,
            1-352, 1-369, 1-400, 1-506,
            1-509, 1-512, 1-513, 2-235–
            2-237, 2-239, 2-240, 3-662,
            3-664–3-666
        $GABA_B$, 1-257, 1-506
γ-hydroxybutyric acid (GBH), 2-486, 3-
    215, 3-216
    liquid ecstasy, 2-486, 3-215
γ-secretase, 2-389, 2-390
delta-opioid receptor, 2-422, 2-425
kappa-opioid receptor, 2-420, 2-422, 2-
    425
mu-opioid receptor, 1-286, 1-287,
        2-236, 2-420–2-422, 2-424,
        2-425, 3-460, 3-476, 3-645

    antagonist, 2-315
Álamo, Cecilio, 3-767, 3-771
Étienne Bonnot de Condillac, 1-86
Claviceps purpurea, see rye ergot
The Mysteries of Opium Reveal'd, see
    opium
nicocanino, 1-119
"ecstasy" vegetables, 2-463
'ezhane' sickness, 3-430
L-DOPA, 2-45, 3-504, 3-773
1-(1-phenylcyclohexyl) piperidine, 3-22
1-aminocyclopropanecarboxylic acid
    (ACPC), 3-642, 3-643, 3-667
2,5-dimethoxy-4-(n)-propylthio-
    phenethylamine (2C-T-7),
    2-355, 2-480
2-amino-6-(trifluoromethoxy) ben-
    zothiazole, *see* riluzole
2-aminophosphoheptanoic acid, 3-642
3,4-methylenedioxy-N-ethylam-
    phetamine (MDEA), 2-480
3,4-methylenedioxyamphetamine
    (MDA), 2-355, 2-480, 2-481,
    2-537
3,4-methylenedioxymethamphetamine
    (MDMA), 2-355–2-357, 2-480,
    2-481, 2-537, 3-54, 3-200,
    3-201, 3-215, 3-774
3277 RP, *see* promethazine
4-methyl-2,5-dimethoxyamphetamine
    (DOM; STP), 2-355, 2-480,
    2-486
5-HIAA, *see* 5-hydroxyindoleacetic acid
5-HT, *see* serotonin
$5\text{-}HT_{1A}$, *see* serotonin
$5\text{-}HT_{1B}$, *see* serotonin
$5\text{-}HT_{1D}$, *see* serotonin
$5\text{-}HT_{1}$, *see* serotonin
$5\text{-}HT_{2A}$, *see* serotonin
$5\text{-}HT_{2B}$, *see* serotonin
$5\text{-}HT_{2C}$, *see* serotonin
$5\text{-}HT_{2}$, *see* serotonin
$5\text{-}HT_{3}$, *see* serotonin

5-HT$_4$, *see* serotonin

5-HT$_6$, *see* serotonin

5-HT$_7$, *see* serotonin

5-MeO-DMT

    5-methoxy-DMT, 2-449

5-hydroxy-tryptophan, *see* 5-hydroxytryptophan (5-HTP)

5-hydroxyindoleacetic acid, 1-465, 1-481, 2-144

    5-HIAA, 1-465, 1-481–1-484, 1-486, 1-493, 2-144, 2-152

5-hydroxytryptophan (5-HTP), 1-466, 1-483, 1-484, 2-144, 2-152, 2-156

    5-hydroxy-tryptophan, 3-771

5-methoxy-DMT, *see* 5-MeO-DMT

8-OH-DPAT, 1-396

9-OH-risperidone, *see* risperidone

9-hydroxyrisperidone, *see* paliperidone

A

A$_2$, *see* adenosine

Abbas, Haly, 1-47, 3-125, 3-439

abdomen, 2-307

abecarnil, 3-663

abnormalities, *see* abnormality

abnormality, 1-xiv, 1-10, 1-249, 1-250, 1-254, 1-269, 1-288, 1-442, 1-446, 1-451, 1-481, 2-96, 2-285, 2-399, 2-401, 2-409, 3-334, 3-335, 3-432, 3-471, 3-517, 3-520, 3-715

abortion, 3-77, 3-125, 3-496

abscess, 3-439

absorption, 1-123, 1-135, 1-361, 1-363, 1-369, 1-378, 1-380, 1-442, 2-59, 2-137, 2-254, 2-283, 2-360, 2-546, 2-558, 3-156, 3-467, 3-585

Abstem, *see* disulfiram

abstinence, 1-406, 2-35, 2-286, 2-311–2-313, 2-405, 2-490, 2-496–2-498, 2-559–2-561, 3-186

abstinence syndrome, 2-285, 2-405, 2-453, 2-497, 2-498, 2-522, 3-68, 3-207, 3-215, *see also* withdrawal syndrome

Abstinyl, *see* disulfiram

AC, *see* adenylyl cyclase (AC)

acamprosate, 2-312, 2-313

    calcium acetylhomotaurine, 2-312

acceptor of action's result, 1-217, 1-220, 1-224–1-227, 1-229

ACE, *see* angiotensin-converting enzyme (ACE)

acetal, 1-129, 1-146

acetanilide, 1-130, 1-141, 1-151

acetaphenolacetic amidophenol, 1-150

acetazolamide, 1-335

acetic acid, 1-329, 1-346, 2-88, 2-507

acetic anhydride, 3-54

acetic ethers, 1-119

acetol, 3-796

acetone, 1-134, 1-139, 1-148, 1-149, 1-365, 2-79, 2-271

acetone diethyl sulfone, 1-149

acetophenone, 1-127, 1-134, 1-149, 2-76

    Hypnone, 1-127, 1-134, 1-139, 1-140, 1-149, 1-151

acetylation, 1-252, 1-384, 3-553, 3-565, 3-566

acetylcholine (ACh), 1-162, 1-205, 1-235, 1-243, 1-254, 1-268, 1-284, 1-451, 2-14, 2-15, 2-17, 2-158, 2-382–2-384, 2-386, 2-464, 3-5, 3-570, 3-596, 3-598, 3-600, 3-610, 3-653, 3-664, 3-714, 3-715, 3-723, 3-747, 3-771

acetylcholine shock, 3-384

acetylcholinesterase (AChE), 2-383, 2-448

acetylmethadone

    L-acetylmethadone, 2-514

acetylsalicylic acid, 2-6
    Aspirin, 2-6, 3-278
ACh, see acetylcholine (ACh)
Achúcarro, Nicolás, 3-712, 3-714, 3-744
AChE, see acetylcholinesterase (AChE)
acidosis, 1-335
Ackerknecht, Erwin H., 1-100, 1-101, 1-
        105, 1-107
aconitase, 3-563
aconite, see aconitine
aconitine, 1-119, 1-144, 1-151, 3-492,
        see also monkshood
    aconite, 1-119, 1-124, 1-130, 1-141
    crystallized aconite, 1-144
Acosta, Cristóbal, 2-517
ACP-104, see norclozapine
ACPC, see 1-aminocyclopropanecar-
        boxylic acid (ACPC)
acquired immunodeficiency syndrome
        (HIV/AIDS), 1-50, 1-359,
        2-315, 2-353, 2-418, 2-471,
        2-514, 2-521, 3-42, 3-52,
        3-199, 3-252, 3-255, 3-569,
        3-571, 3-584
    dementia, 3-560
    epidemic, 2-309
Actaea racemosa, 2-328
ACTH, see adrenocorticotropic hor-
        mone (ACTH)
actin, 1-259, 3-563
actinomycin D, 1-226
action potential, 1-186, 1-205, 1-240, 1-
        242, 1-260, 3-600
Action T4, 3-94, 3-95
active transport, 1-264
acute mania, 1-131, 1-379, 2-185, 2-192,
        2-193, 2-211, 3-310, 3-363
acylation, 1-252
Adam,   see   MDMA   (methylene-
        dioxymethamphetamine)
Adams, Roger, 2-271, 2-522
adatanserin, 1-326
addiction, 1-111, 1-112, 1-136, 1-407,

        1-409,   1-527–1-531,   2-207,
        2-281,   2-299,   2-305–2-308,
        2-310,   2-315,   2-418,   2-419,
        2-472,   2-508,   2-510,   2-511,
        2-522, 2-560, 3-39, 3-41, 3-69,
        3-137,   3-186,   3-190,   3-205,
        3-293,   3-316,   3-329,   3-385,
        3-464,   3-493,   3-496,   3-552,
        3-564, 3-566, 3-645, 3-775
    heroin, 2-308, 2-475, 2-514
Addison's disease, 1-331
adenosine
    receptor, 2-354
        A$_2$, 3-660
adenosine diphosphate
    ADP, 1-252
adenosine triphosphate, 1-252, 1-447
    ATP, 1-252, 1-447, 1-466, 3-563
adenylate cyclase, see adenylyl cyclase
        (AC)
adenylyl cyclase, 1-254, 1-255, 1-257, 1-
        285, 1-287, 3-600
adenylyl cyclase (AC), 1-254, 3-512–3-
        514, 3-600, 3-634
Ader, Robert, 2-398
Adler, Alfred, 3-715
Adonis vernalis, 1-130, 1-160
ADP, see adenosine diphosphate
adrenal cortex, 1-484
adrenal insufficiency, 1-331
adrenal medulla, 1-488
adrenergic, 1-205, 1-242, 1-243, 1-268,
        1-280,   1-319,   1-327,   1-343,
        1-346,   1-350,   1-466,   1-469,
        1-470, 1-484, 1-485, 1-488–1-
        490, 2-45, 2-46, 2-96, 2-150,
        2-152,   2-159,   2-177,   2-309,
        2-310,   2-351,   3-453,   3-457,
        3-512,   3-517,   3-562,   3-583,
        3-594,   3-596,   3-598,   3-606,
        3-630,   3-649,   3-771,   3-772,
        3-774
adrenergic receptor

α, 2-168

α_1, 1-259, 1-312, 1-343, 1-400, 1-488, 2-96, 2-150, 2-159, 2-175, 2-177, 3-299, 3-662, 3-663, 3-665

α_2, 1-257, 1-312, 1-327, 1-357, 1-400, 1-484, 1-488–1-490, 2-46, 2-96, 2-150, 2-159, 2-174–2-176, 3-459, 3-474, 3-630, 3-662, 3-663, 3-771, 3-774

β, 1-243, 1-257, 1-284, 1-285, 1-488–1-490, 2-152, 2-159, 3-514, 3-630, 3-642

β_1, 1-488

β_2, 1-255, 1-346, 3-583, 3-655

β_3, 1-488

adrenocorticotropic hormone (ACTH), 1-221, 1-222, 1-226, 1-262, 1-399, 1-484, 1-514, 3-418, 3-635, 3-640, 3-642, 3-775

Adrian, Edgar D., 1-205

affective disorders, 1-295, 1-399, 2-45, 2-206, 2-402, 2-562, 3-140, 3-303, 3-305, 3-306, 3-354, 3-367, 3-398, 3-511, 3-626, 3-633, 3-660, 3-666, 3-773, 3-775

afferent, 1-217, 1-229, 1-409

aggressiveness, 2-35, 2-37, 2-366, 2-557, 3-108, 3-205, 3-207, 3-215, 3-467

Aghili, Mohamed Hosin, 3-125

agnosia, 2-381

agomelatine, 3-647

agoraphobia, 1-14, 1-505, 2-160, 3-621

agranulocytosis, 1-312, 1-358, 2-59, 2-285, 3-61, 3-67, 3-132, 3-298, 3-299, 3-474

Agustín, Fray Farfán, 2-497

Ahlquist, Raymon P., 1-171, 1-237

AJ-76, 3-651

ajmalicine, 2-30

ajmaline, 2-30, 2-31

ajmalinine, 2-30

akathisia, 2-17, 2-39, 2-45, 2-60, 2-366

al'Abbas, Ali ibn, see Abbas, Haly

Al-Abbas-al-Majusi, Ali Ebn, see Abbas, Haly

Al-Hakem II, Caliph, 3-732

Alarcón, Renato D., 3-729

albinism, 3-430

albuminuria, 1-144

alchemy, 1-64, 1-65, 2-438, 2-439, 2-449, 3-230

alcohol, 1-119, 1-134, 1-138, 1-140, 1-159, 1-221, 1-294, 1-305, 1-317, 1-377, 1-406, 1-410, 1-505, 2-88, 2-113, 2-208, 2-220, 2-265, 2-271, 2-276, 2-305, 2-306, 2-310–2-316, 2-341, 2-363, 2-415, 2-417, 2-438, 2-451, 2-452, 2-458, 2-471, 2-476, 2-477, 2-486, 2-489–2-492, 2-494–2-498, 2-507, 2-513, 2-514, 2-519, 2-522, 2-529, 2-550, 2-557, 2-558, 2-562, 2-563, 3-48, 3-187–3-189, 3-196, 3-201, 3-202, 3-204–3-208, 3-214–3-216, 3-218, 3-285, 3-293, 3-433, 3-434, 3-437, 3-494, 3-524, 3-563, 3-564, 3-652, 3-662, 3-665, 3-666

alcohol dehydrogenase (ADH), 3-561

alcoholic hallucinosis, 3-749

alcoholic intoxication, 3-497

alcoholism, 1-9, 1-134, 1-149, 2-160, 2-161, 2-305–2-307, 2-311–2-313, 2-348, 2-401, 2-489, 2-494, 2-496, 2-497, 2-524, 2-536, 3-68, 3-91, 3-207, 3-208, 3-329, 3-434, 3-495, 3-723, 3-789, 3-801

Aldini, Giovanni, 3-344

Alexander Shulgin, 2-481

Alguacil, Luis F., 1-xxviii
alizarin, 2-58
alkaloid, 1-72, 1-121, 1-129, 1-147, 1-155, 1-307, 1-346, 2-29–2-32, 2-34, 2-266, 2-328, 2-361, 2-442, 2-445–2-447, 2-453–2-456, 2-461, 2-464, 2-475, 2-477–2-479, 2-526, 2-545, 3-189, 3-198, 3-661, 3-764
alkylation, 2-295
Allegron, *see* nortriptyline
allergic alveolitis, 3-64
allergy, 2-398, 3-6, 3-7
ALLO, *see* allopregnanolone
allobarbital
    Dial, 1-156, 1-158, 1-160, 2-275
    diallylbarbituric acid, 1-156
allopregnanolone, 3-665, 3-666
    ALLO, 3-666
allosteric, 1-268, 1-284, 1-323, 2-384, 2-387, 3-509, 3-599, 3-600, 3-610, 3-658, 3-665
allyl tribromide, 1-146, 1-147
alnespirone, 2-247
    DU-125530, 2-247
    S-15535, 2-247
alopecia, 3-466
Alosetron, 1-319
alpha 2-adrenergic agonist, 2-309
alpha-methyl-p-tyrosine   (AMPT), 1-488, 2-16
alphaxolone, 2-279
alpidem, 2-238
alprazolam, 2-233, 3-144, 3-217, 3-476, 3-666, 3-668
    Xanax, 2-233
alternative splicing, 1-254, 1-281, 1-283, 1-286
Altschule, Mark D., 2-35
Alurate, *see* aprobarbital
Alzheimer's Disease, 1-169, 1-263, 1-289, 2-355, 2-381, 2-384, 2-388, 3-546, 3-552, 3-560–3-562, 3-564, 3-604, 3-607, 3-653–3-655, 3-795
    dementia, 2-366
Alzheimer, Alois, 3-712, 3-714
Amanita muscaria, 1-62, 1-130, 1-322, 2-433, 2-464, 3-185
amantadine, 2-310
    Symmetrel, 2-310
American Indians, 2-486
American Medical Association (AMA), 1-160, 2-8, 2-269, 2-494, 2-510, 2-523, 3-88, 3-126, 3-143
American Pharmaceutical Association, 2-281, 3-202
American   Pharmacists   Association (APhA), 3-202
American Pharmacopeia, *see* United States Pharmacopeia
American   Psychiatric   Association (APA), 1-25, 2-26, 2-42, 2-197, 2-209, 2-522, 3-136, 3-180, 3-239, 3-243, 3-247, 3-322, 3-350, 3-402, 3-462, 3-522
American Psychological Association, 2-522
amfepramone, 3-67, 3-68
amidothymidine, 1-226
amineptine, 2-135, 3-68
amino acid metabolism, 3-362
aminoglutethimide, 3-640
Aminophylline, *see also* theophylline
Amiot, R.P. Jean-Joseph-Marie, 1-67
amisulpride, 2-98
Amital, *see* amobarbital
amitriptyline, 1-337, 1-339, 1-357, 1-361, 1-382, 2-13, 2-110, 2-112, 2-113, 2-129, 2-130, 2-135, 2-137, 2-138, 2-144, 2-146, 2-156, 2-159, 2-171, 2-172, 2-174, 2-175, 3-132, 3-314, 3-448, 3-450–3-457, 3-460, 3-462, 3-464, 3-645, 3-772

Elavil, 2-130

Saroten, 2-130

ammonia, 1-73, 1-142, 1-146, 1-147, 1-339, 2-440, 2-442

ammonium, 1-129

ammonium bromide, 1-140

amnesia, 1-509, 2-236, 2-282, 2-557, 3-64, 3-65, 3-215, 3-346, 3-439, 3-499, 3-662, 3-663, 3-773

amobarbital, 1-506, 2-272, 2-278, 2-279, 2-281, 2-282, 2-285, 2-286

Amital, 1-160

Amytal, 1-506, 2-272, 3-496

amonol, 1-146

amoxapine, 1-339, 2-94, 2-110, 2-135

AMPA receptor, 1-253, 2-387, 3-644, 3-658

ampakine, 3-658

Ampalex, *see* CX-516

amperometry, 1-367

amphetamine, 1-162, 1-242, 1-341, 1-347, 1-356, 1-395, 1-401, 1-404, 1-405, 1-408, 1-409, 1-469, 1-470, 1-472, 1-489, 1-492, 1-528–1-530, 2-4, 2-17, 2-81, 2-84, 2-94, 2-95, 2-108, 2-348–2-350, 2-353, 2-463, 2-480, 2-523, 2-524, 2-533, 3-23, 3-199, 3-200, 3-418, 3-419, 3-498, 3-504, 3-563, 3-566, 3-652, 3-656, 3-765, 3-773

Benzedrine, 2-479, 2-523

schizophrenia, 1-405

amphetamine derivatives, 1-479, 2-282, 2-349, 2-354, 2-355

amphetamine-type anorexic stimulants, 3-471

amphetamines, 1-xxiv, 1-xxv, 1-409, 2-4, 2-12, 2-44, 2-107, 2-220, 2-267, 2-311, 2-347, 2-349–2-357, 2-479, 2-480, 2-523–2-525, 2-529, 3-54, 3-55, 3-189, 3-199, 3-200, 3-205, 3-209, 3-210, 3-491, 3-498, 3-658, 3-763, 3-764, 3-770–3-773

AMPT, *see* alpha-methyl-p-tyrosine (AMPT)

amulet, 3-128

amygdophenine, 1-146, 1-151

amyl nitrite, 1-151, 2-486

amyl valerianate, 1-148

amylene, 1-129, 1-148

amylene chloral, *see* dormiol

amylene hydrate, 1-158, 2-276

amyloid peptide, 2-390

amyloid precursor protein (APP), 1-290, 2-389, 2-390

amyotrophic lateral sclerosis, 3-559, 3-603, 3-604, 3-643

Amytal, *see* amobarbital

anabolic steroids, 2-160

Anafranil, *see* clomipramine

analeptic, 1-162, 1-345, 1-349, 2-347, 2-524, 2-535

analgene, 1-151

analgesia, 2-285, 2-354, 2-422, 2-432, 3-229, 3-447, 3-456, 3-459, 3-460, 3-473

analgesic, 1-123, 1-129, 1-134, 1-135, 1-139, 1-141, 1-142, 1-146, 1-147, 1-150, 1-152, 1-154, 1-158, 1-286, 1-305, 1-316, 1-341, 1-350, 1-528, 2-3, 2-32, 2-61, 2-75–2-77, 2-79, 2-111, 2-176, 2-206, 2-308, 2-414, 2-416, 2-417, 2-419, 2-420, 2-423, 2-431, 2-439, 2-443, 2-453, 2-475, 2-505, 2-506, 2-510, 2-511, 2-514, 2-517, 2-521, 3-9, 3-54, 3-189, 3-193, 3-213, 3-216, 3-362, 3-374, 3-417, 3-448, 3-450, 3-451, 3-453–3-457, 3-459–3-461, 3-466, 3-473–3-476,

3-771–3-773
anaphrodistic, 1-144
anastomosis, 1-191, 1-194, 1-201
anatomy, 1-8, 1-10, 1-11, 1-28, 1-64, 1-183, 1-184, 1-194, 2-82, 2-441, 2-521, 3-715
Ancien Régime, 1-4, 1-75, 1-87, 3-711, 3-717, 3-718
Anderson, N. Leigh, 3-553
Anderson, Norman G., 3-553
androgens, 2-405
anemia, 1-127, 1-131, 1-141, 1-143–1-145, 1-148, 1-149, 2-494, 2-510
  aplastic, 2-204, 3-66
  hemolytic, 3-64
anesthesia, 1-111, 1-134, 1-139, 1-149, 1-151, 1-220, 1-305, 1-349, 1-420, 1-512, 2-7, 2-55, 2-60, 2-221, 2-225, 2-253, 2-254, 2-258, 2-278, 2-279, 2-286, 2-343, 2-355, 2-431, 2-432, 2-437, 2-442–2-445, 2-447, 3-6, 3-9, 3-22, 3-24, 3-214, 3-216, 3-353, 3-472, 3-473
  general, 1-305, 2-266, 2-445, 2-447, 3-352
  intravenous, 2-272, 2-278
  local, 2-445, 2-478
  neuroleptanesthesia, 1-305
  regional, 2-445, 2-529
  spinal, 2-478
anesthetic, 1-110, 1-132, 1-134, 1-147, 1-148, 1-305, 1-416, 1-418, 1-420, 2-61, 2-65, 2-222, 2-254, 2-258, 2-265, 2-279, 2-285, 2-286, 2-338, 2-355, 2-437, 2-440, 2-442, 2-445, 2-448, 2-516, 2-525, 2-529, 2-557, 3-22, 3-23, 3-216, 3-349, 3-350, 3-352, 3-362, 3-437, 3-475, 3-507
Anexate, see mefenorex

Angel Dust, see phencyclidine
angina pectoris, 2-510
angioedema, 3-466, 3-467
angiotensin II, 1-222, 1-400
angiotensin-converting enzyme (ACE), 1-294, 3-307
Angst, Jules, 2-95
anhydroglucochloral, 1-148
animal model, 1-xxvi, 1-176, 1-178, 1-179, 1-284, 1-369, 1-393, 1-394, 1-397, 1-399, 1-401, 1-403–1-405, 1-407, 1-485, 1-508, 1-530, 1-531, 2-93–2-95, 2-154–2-156, 2-203, 2-208, 2-246, 2-369, 2-370, 2-383, 2-387, 2-389, 3-22, 3-25, 3-27, 3-363, 3-364, 3-521, 3-526, 3-563, 3-639, 3-645, 3-664, 3-666, 3-668, 3-772, 3-773
aniracetam, 3-644
anodyne, 1-132, 2-332, 2-507, 2-519
Anokhin, P.K., 1-219, 1-220
Anokhin, Petr K., 1-214
anorectic, 1-343, 3-660, 3-771
anorexia nervosa, 2-401
Anslinger, Harry J., 3-185
Antabuse, see disulfiram
antagonist, 1-238, 1-245, 1-314, 1-319, 1-462, 1-471, 1-472, 1-481, 1-484, 1-485, 1-492, 2-81, 2-96–2-98, 2-153, 2-208, 2-247, 2-308–2-310, 2-313, 2-386, 2-420, 3-366, 3-508, 3-562, 3-563, 3-599, 3-609, 3-640, 3-641, 3-644, 3-646–3-648, 3-652–3-655, 3-659, 3-660, 3-665, 3-667, 3-668, 3-771
anterior, 1-48, 1-52, 1-408, 1-444, 1-451, 3-401, 3-507, 3-601, 3-735, 3-785
anterior pituitary, 2-397
anti/insomnia, 1-147
anti/nervous medicines, 1-146

anti-aggression, 2-364

anti-aggressive, 2-367

anti-agonistic, 2-370

anti-alcohol, 2-497

anti-alcohol serum, 2-497

anti-anxiety, 2-236, 2-238

anti-apoptotic, 1-265

anti-asthmatic, 2-479

anti-depressant, 2-311

anti-doping, 3-200

anti-epilepsy, 2-311

anti-immobility, 2-156

anti-infective, 3-7, 3-642

anti-inflammatory, 1-123, 2-409, 2-423,
    3-448, 3-646

anti-mania, 1-xxiv

anti-maniacal, 1-21

anti-nausea, 2-480

anti-neurasthenic, 1-152, 1-153

anti-obesity, 3-69

anti-obsessive, 2-33

anti-Semitic, 3-89

anti-serum, 1-222

anti-spasmodic, 1-148, 2-479

antiadrenergic, 2-94, 3-299

antibiotic, 1-418, 2-5, 2-11, 2-220,
    2-315, 2-339, 2-534, 2-535,
    3-4, 3-5, 3-8, 3-280

antibodies, 1-280, 1-283, 1-510, 2-391,
    2-402, 3-560, 3-566, 3-570

anticholinergic, 1-312, 1-318, 1-326, 1-
    336, 1-382, 2-79, 2-85, 2-86, 2-
    94, 2-111, 2-136, 2-144, 2-159,
    3-299, 3-365, 3-463, 3-466, 3-
    499

anticonvulsant, 1-123, 1-233, 1-269,
    1-323, 1-328–1-331, 1-333–
    1-335, 1-375, 1-376, 1-378,
    1-509, 2-4, 2-32, 2-111, 2-189–
    2-191, 2-193–2-197, 2-203,
    2-204, 2-206, 2-208, 2-210,
    2-211, 2-233, 2-236, 2-261,
    2-267, 2-270, 2-276, 2-278,
    2-279, 2-283, 2-285, 2-286,
    2-294, 2-296, 2-313, 2-367,
    2-518, 2-521, 2-523, 2-555,
    2-561, 3-22, 3-24, 3-25, 3-27,
    3-277, 3-447, 3-605, 3-662,
    3-664, 3-685, 3-771

anticonvulsive hypothesis, 3-348

antidepressant, 1-ix, 1-xxv, 1-xxvii, 1-
    22, 1-176–1-178, 1-207, 1-241,
    1-242, 1-249, 1-250, 1-253,
    1-257, 1-269, 1-314, 1-327,
    1-335–1-337,   1-339–1-341,
    1-343, 1-352, 1-356, 1-357,
    1-359–1-365,   1-370,   1-375,
    1-377,   1-380–1-385,   1-395,
    1-399, 1-406, 1-415, 1-419–
    1-421, 1-423, 1-429, 1-441,
    1-447, 1-448, 1-450, 1-479,
    1-480,   1-482–1-488,   1-490–
    1-492,   1-494–1-496,   1-513,
    1-514, 2-3, 2-13, 2-15, 2-16,
    2-41, 2-45, 2-94, 2-105, 2-107–
    2-115, 2-125, 2-128, 2-130,
    2-132,   2-133,   2-135–2-138,
    2-141, 2-142, 2-144, 2-146,
    2-148,   2-152–2-158,   2-160,
    2-167, 2-168, 2-176, 2-197,
    2-205–2-207,   2-225,   2-245–
    2-247, 2-249, 2-285, 2-349,
    2-351, 2-353, 2-367, 2-405,
    2-407–2-409,   2-448,   2-458,
    2-477, 2-515, 2-522, 2-538,
    3-8, 3-11, 3-12, 3-24, 3-64,
    3-67–3-69, 3-81, 3-82, 3-113,
    3-114,   3-130–3-132,   3-140,
    3-144, 3-180, 3-218, 3-226,
    3-238, 3-239, 3-245–3-247,
    3-250, 3-251, 3-277–3-279,
    3-283, 3-298, 3-305, 3-306,
    3-310, 3-312–3-315, 3-327,
    3-331, 3-332, 3-336, 3-352,
    3-353, 3-365–3-368, 3-374,
    3-386–3-388, 3-447, 3-448,

3-450–3-457, 3-459–3-461, 3-463–3-468, 3-471, 3-474, 3-504, 3-509, 3-510, 3-512, 3-514, 3-516–3-518, 3-520, 3-521, 3-523, 3-525, 3-562, 3-584, 3-594, 3-606, 3-610, 3-625, 3-626, 3-628–3-631, 3-633–3-637, 3-639, 3-640, 3-642–3-648, 3-652, 3-654, 3-662, 3-664–3-669, 3-765, 3-769–3-774, 3-798, 3-800

antidopaminergic, 2-84, 2-85, 2-94, 3-334

antiemetic, 1-314, 1-318, 1-321, 1-421, 2-69, 2-176, 2-521, 3-49, 3-472, 3-473, 3-646

antiepileptic, 1-126, 1-146, 1-328, 1-335, 1-349, 1-364, 1-376, 1-378, 1-379, 1-506, 2-195, 2-203, 2-204, 2-206, 2-208–2-210, 2-277, 2-278, 3-84, 3-181, 3-460, 3-604, 3-664, 3-667, 3-800

Antiethyl, *see* disulfiram

antiflatulent, 2-517

antihistaminic, 1-307, 1-308, 1-311, 1-357, 2-7, 2-12, 2-56–2-58, 2-60, 2-61, 2-64, 2-65, 2-71, 2-82, 2-126, 2-219, 3-365, 3-467, 3-475

antihypertensive, 1-307, 1-340, 1-341, 1-418, 2-10, 2-23, 2-40, 3-307

antihysteric, 1-146, 1-147

antimalarial, 1-307, 2-58

antimanic, 1-ix, 1-380, 2-86, 2-87, 2-189, 2-191–2-194, 2-196, 2-197, 2-203, 2-205, 2-207, 2-208, 2-210, 3-306, 3-504, 3-512, 3-520, 3-625, 3-755

antinervine, 1-151

antineuralgic, 1-134, 1-142, 1-144, 1-146, 1-148

antinociceptive, 2-425, 3-476, 3-646

antiparasitic, 1-123, 1-169

antiparkinson, 1-311, 2-58, 2-111, 2-353, 3-652

antiphospholipid syndrome, 2-402

antiprotozoal, 3-6

antipruritic, 3-467

antipsychiatry, 1-22, 3-84, 3-231, 3-232, 3-283, 3-322, 3-347

antipsychotic, 1-ix, 1-xvi, 1-xxvii, 1-168, 1-177, 1-178, 1-207, 1-238, 1-241, 1-242, 1-245, 1-249, 1-277, 1-307, 1-309, 1-311, 1-312, 1-314, 1-321, 1-339, 1-358–1-364, 1-369, 1-375, 1-383, 1-385, 1-395, 1-404–1-406, 1-415, 1-441, 1-445, 1-446, 1-448, 1-449, 1-468, 1-471, 1-472, 1-479, 2-13, 2-23, 2-27, 2-33, 2-34, 2-39, 2-40, 2-42, 2-45, 2-46, 2-55, 2-56, 2-71, 2-75, 2-82, 2-86, 2-88, 2-93–2-100, 2-127, 2-129, 2-158, 2-184, 2-192, 2-194, 2-206, 2-208, 2-210, 2-211, 2-225, 2-230–2-232, 2-245, 2-365, 2-366, 2-401, 2-407, 2-514, 3-11, 3-61, 3-66, 3-69, 3-70, 3-82, 3-130, 3-132–3-136, 3-174, 3-180, 3-181, 3-218, 3-227, 3-234, 3-238, 3-239, 3-244, 3-247, 3-249, 3-250, 3-252, 3-277, 3-278, 3-283, 3-284, 3-298–3-300, 3-306, 3-308–3-310, 3-312, 3-316, 3-334, 3-364, 3-367, 3-368, 3-447, 3-472–3-475, 3-503, 3-504, 3-506–3-508, 3-520, 3-521, 3-523, 3-525, 3-567, 3-585, 3-594, 3-612, 3-625, 3-626, 3-648–3-662, 3-685, 3-761, 3-766, 3-773, 3-798, 3-800

antipyretic, 1-123, 1-140, 1-147, 2-494,

2-516, 2-523, 3-418
antipyretics, 1-130, 1-146, 2-6
antipyrine, 1-130, 1-141, 1-144, 1-146, 1-151, 1-159
antiretrovirals, 3-255
antirheumatic, 1-147
antisepsis, 2-431
antiserum, 1-222
antispasmodic, 1-73, 1-90, 1-97, 1-119, 1-123, 1-129, 1-143, 1-146, 1-157, 2-448, 3-463
antisuicidal, 2-193, 3-311, 3-314, 3-316
antithermal, 1-146
antitubercular, 1-357, 1-419, 2-106
antitussive, 1-311, 2-111, 2-355, 2-523, 2-537
Antoine-Chantin Hospital, 2-61
Antonio, Marco, 2-438
anus, 1-122, 2-436, 3-345
anxiety, 1-ix, 1-x, 1-xxiv, 1-109, 1-120, 1-162, 1-319, 1-322, 1-323, 1-326, 1-327, 1-337, 1-352, 1-357, 1-394–1-397, 1-399, 1-421, 1-422, 1-485, 1-493–1-495, 1-505, 1-506, 1-508–1-514, 2-4, 2-7, 2-11, 2-12, 2-35, 2-39, 2-59, 2-67, 2-105, 2-109, 2-111, 2-115, 2-138, 2-155, 2-157, 2-159, 2-173, 2-176, 2-203, 2-207, 2-210, 2-220, 2-222, 2-223, 2-225, 2-230–2-234, 2-236, 2-237, 2-239, 2-240, 2-246–2-249, 2-293, 2-310, 2-357, 2-361, 2-363, 2-365, 2-366, 2-368, 2-370, 2-404, 2-408, 2-454, 2-513, 2-519, 2-535, 2-549, 2-555, 2-556, 2-562, 3-5, 3-64, 3-68, 3-82, 3-140, 3-180, 3-250, 3-282, 3-285, 3-292, 3-293, 3-305, 3-306, 3-308, 3-309, 3-315, 3-316, 3-325, 3-331–3-333, 3-344, 3-346,
3-372–3-374, 3-385, 3-387, 3-389, 3-406, 3-417, 3-418, 3-420, 3-438, 3-439, 3-447, 3-453, 3-467, 3-471, 3-475, 3-476, 3-523, 3-594, 3-608, 3-611, 3-621, 3-641, 3-654, 3-660, 3-662, 3-664–3-669, 3-738, 3-747, 3-771, 3-775, 3-793
anxiety disorder, 2-207, 2-210, 2-232, 2-246, 2-248, 2-562, 3-82, 3-315, 3-406
anxiolytic, 1-269, 1-323, 1-326, 1-362, 1-394–1-397, 1-485, 1-506–1-512, 2-13, 2-33, 2-86, 2-232, 2-236, 2-238–2-240, 2-245–2-249, 2-366, 2-555, 3-10, 3-25, 3-130, 3-140, 3-217, 3-306, 3-315, 3-447, 3-456, 3-466, 3-626, 3-646, 3-654, 3-658, 3-662–3-668, 3-800
aphasia, 2-381
apnea, 1-156, 2-296, 2-354
Apocynaceae, 2-24
Apolisina, 1-146
apomorphine, 1-131, 1-132, 1-489, 1-492, 2-4, 2-17, 2-81, 2-84, 2-88, 2-94, 2-95, 2-97, 2-146, 2-305, 2-306, 2-308, 2-328, 3-773
apomorphine chloride, 1-146
Aponal, see doxepin
apoptosis, 1-257, 1-265, 3-570, 3-612
APP, see amyloid precursor protein (APP)
appendix, 3-154, 3-156, 3-324
apraxia, 2-381
aprobarbital
    Alurate, 1-160
Aquifoliaceae, 2-456
Araceae, 2-463
arachnoiditis, 1-105
Ardrey, Robert, 3-413

Arfvedson, A., 2-7
argentic salt of barbiturate acid, 2-268
aripiprazole, 2-93, 2-98, 2-99, 2-193, 2-366, 3-506, 3-649
aristol, 1-146
Aristotle, 1-35, 1-43, 1-45, 1-46, 1-74, 1-167, 2-441, 3-379, 3-438, 3-706, 3-732, 3-736
arm, 1-290, 1-405, 1-429, 3-36, 3-37, 3-256, 3-388, 3-621
arrhythmia, 3-68, 3-69
arrhythmias, 2-354, 3-68, 3-69, 3-299
    cardiac, 3-352
arsenate, 1-144
arseniate, 1-159
arsenic, 1-137, 1-140, 1-151, 1-159, 1-377, 2-305, 2-507, 3-492
arsphenamine, 2-339, 3-280
    Salvarsan, 1-236, 2-339, 3-280
arterial sedative, 1-148
arteriosclerosis, 3-135
artery, 1-462, 1-488, 3-787
arthralgia, 3-63
arthritis, 1-137, 1-416
    rheumatoid, 3-324, 3-327
arthritism, 1-137
articulation, 1-196
aryl ethynyl derivatives, 1-334
asafetida, 1-119, 1-129, 1-146, 1-151
asafoetida, 1-73
asaprol, 1-146
asarone, 2-463
Aschenbrandt, Theodor, 2-527
asenapine, 2-98, 2-193, 3-653
asphyxia, 1-123, 1-141
Aspidosperma quebracho, 1-130
Aspirin, see acetylsalicylic acid
association analysis, 1-289
asthma, 1-121, 1-127, 1-150, 1-291, 2-56, 2-58, 2-247, 2-348, 2-354, 2-398, 2-448, 2-498, 2-519, 2-521, 2-523, 2-527, 2-528, 3-6
Astier, P., 1-153

Ataractan, see azacyclonol
ataxia, 1-334, 1-421, 2-557, 3-547, 3-607
Atharvaveda, see Ayurveda
atherosclerosis, 1-152, 3-787
atorvastatin, 3-22
    Lipitor, 3-22
ATP, see adenosine triphosphate
Atrium, see tetrabamate
Atropa belladonna, see Belladonna (Atropa belladonna)
Atropa mandragora, see Mandrake
atrophy, 2-154, 3-639, 3-666, 3-667, 3-669
atropine, 1-118, 1-119, 1-121, 1-124, 1-130, 1-151, 1-155, 1-234, 2-38, 2-266, 2-305, 2-306, 2-328, 2-361, 2-434, 2-445, 2-448, 2-449, 3-499, see also Mandrake, Belladonna
    atropine coma, 3-384
attention deficit hyperactivity disorder (ADHD), 2-350, 2-357, 2-525, 2-530, 2-531, 2-533, 3-25, 3-69, 3-83, 3-244–3-247, 3-402, 3-403, 3-417, 3-418, 3-464, 3-655
atypical, 1-xvi, 1-242, 1-259, 1-294, 1-295, 1-314, 1-321, 1-358, 1-405, 1-406, 1-445, 1-446, 1-448, 1-449, 1-471, 1-472, 2-12, 2-65, 2-75, 2-82, 2-88, 2-93, 2-96–2-99, 2-110, 2-115, 2-152, 2-158, 2-167, 2-185, 2-206, 2-208, 2-309, 2-366, 3-61, 3-132, 3-133, 3-218, 3-234, 3-244, 3-247, 3-250, 3-278, 3-299, 3-308, 3-312, 3-316, 3-331, 3-332, 3-334, 3-335, 3-420, 3-472, 3-474, 3-475, 3-506, 3-508, 3-612, 3-626, 3-636, 3-648–3-650, 3-652–3-654, 3-658, 3-659, 3-661, 3-772

atypicality, 2-93, 2-95, 2-96, 2-98, 2-99, 3-650

Aubert-Roche, Louis Rémy, 2-518

auditory, 1-225, 2-273, 2-547, 3-206

August Pi i Sunyer, 3-757

Aurelianus, Caelius, 1-40–1-42, 2-363

autoantibodies, 2-402

autonomic nervous system, 1-169, 1-205, 1-233, 1-238, 2-7, 2-58, 2-114, 2-219, 2-220, 2-222, 2-386, 3-5, 3-595

Aversan, see disulfiram

Avicenna, 1-47, 2-415, 2-432, 2-451, 2-456, 2-463, 2-472, 2-506, 2-511, 3-437–3-439, 3-732, 3-738

Axelrod, Julius, 1-205, 1-236, 1-240–1-242, 2-137, 3-510

axon, 1-172, 1-196, 1-199, 1-202, 1-292, 3-563

ayahuasca, 2-445, 2-463, 2-538, 3-797
  Banisteriopsis caapi, 2-463, 2-538, 3-797

Ayd, Frank Joseph, 2-8, 2-40, 2-130, 2-131

Ayurveda, 2-10, 2-23, 2-24, 2-26, 2-27, 2-30, 2-46, 3-432
  Atharvaveda, 2-516, 3-197, 3-377
  Dhanvantari, 2-24
  Kapha, 2-25–2-27
  Pitta, 2-25
  Vata, 2-25, 2-27
  Veda, 2-482, 3-197
  Vedic, 1-322, 2-24, 3-496
  Vishnu, 2-24

azacyclonol, 1-162, 3-762
  Ataractan, 3-762
  Frenquel, 1-162, 3-762

azapirone, 1-324, 1-484, 1-485, 2-246, 2-247

AZD3480, see ispronicline

azidothymidine, 1-226

azotemia, 2-67

B

Babinski, Joseph, 1-15, 3-714

Babinski, Joseph F.F., 3-344

back pain, 2-176

baclofen, 2-209, 2-313, 3-476

Baeyer, Adolf von, 1-119, 1-506, 2-265

Baillarger, Jules, 1-6, 1-105

Bailly, Christian, 2-438

Ballesteros, Luis Rojas, 3-716

balsamic resin, 1-148

Banús, José Sanchis, 3-711, 3-712, 3-722

bang, see cannabis

bangue, see cannabis

Banisteriopsis caapi, see ayahuasca

bapineuzumab, 2-391

barberry, 1-147

barbital, 1-160, 1-352, 1-377, 2-4, 2-268–2-271, 2-281, 2-283, 2-363, 3-662
  barbitone, 1-506, 2-270
  diethylbarbituric acid, 1-156, 1-158, 2-4, 2-229
  diethylmalonyl urea, 1-156
  sodium barbital, 1-160
  Veronal, 1-150, 1-151, 1-156, 1-158, 1-331, 2-4, 2-269, 2-270, 2-281, 2-306, 2-363, 3-496, 3-499

barbitone, see barbital

barbiturate, 1-156, 1-160, 1-329–1-331, 1-349, 1-377, 1-406, 1-422, 1-460, 1-505, 1-506, 2-4, 2-35, 2-58, 2-61, 2-65, 2-194, 2-203, 2-220–2-222, 2-225, 2-229, 2-261, 2-265–2-272, 2-275–2-279, 2-281–2-286, 2-293, 2-329, 2-363, 2-365, 2-520, 2-524, 2-555, 3-54, 3-58, 3-67, 3-87, 3-97, 3-100, 3-210, 3-218, 3-232, 3-349, 3-362, 3-491, 3-495, 3-496, 3-605, 3-662, 3-666

barbituric acid, 1-119, 1-331, 1-505, 2-4, 2-275
    malonyl urea, 1-505
    malonylurea, 2-4, 2-265, 2-267, 2-269
Barbui, Corrado, 2-138
Bardet, Daniel, 1-138, 1-139, 2-278
Bartholow, Robert, 3-88
Baruk, Henri, 3-790, 3-792
Basaglia, Franco, 1-24
Bathelemy, Baron, 1-127
Battie, William, 1-3, 1-84
Baudelaire, Charles, 3-495, 3-497
Bauer, Ida, 1-16
Bayle, Antoine Laurent Jessé, 1-8
Bayle, Antoine-Laurent, 1-105
Beard, George, 1-14
Beaumont, George, 2-133, 3-12, 3-15
Beckett, Arnold, 2-76
Beecher, Henry K., 3-375
Beelzebub, 2-434
beer, 1-xxiii, 1-151, 1-341, 2-110, 2-363, 2-490, 2-492, 2-495, 2-532, 3-204, 3-433, 3-434
befloxatone, 1-341
Bein, Hugo J., 2-30, 2-31
belaperidone, 3-650
Belladonna (Atropa belladonna), 1-42, 1-69, 1-106, 1-108, 1-119, 1-121, 1-122, 1-124, 1-129, 1-137, 1-140, 1-142, 1-151, 1-155, 1-160, 2-265, 2-305, 2-306, 2-359, 2-432–2-434, 2-439, 2-447–2-449, 2-513, 3-185, 3-499
bemegride, 1-331, 1-349
benactyzine, 1-162, 1-326, 3-762
    Suavitil, 3-762
Benadryl, see diphenhydramine (DPH, DHM)
benign, 2-159, 2-204, 2-206, 3-307, 3-309, 3-606
Bentley, W. H., 2-529

Benzedrine, see amphetamine
Benzi, Ugo, 1-50
benzocaine
    norcaine, 2-311
benzodiazepine, 1-395, 1-505–1-507, 1-509, 1-510, 1-514, 2-230, 2-231, 2-233, 2-235–2-240, 2-281, 2-283, 2-293, 2-295–2-297, 2-299, 2-366, 2-555–2-563, 3-137, 3-140, 3-144, 3-214, 3-215, 3-287, 3-298, 3-504, 3-604, 3-605, 3-662–3-666, 3-800
    dependence, 2-559
    discovery, 2-230
    mechanism of action, 2-234
    receptor, 1-369, 1-509–1-511, 2-150, 2-235, 2-245, 2-296, 3-663, 3-665
benzodiazepines, 1-322–1-324, 1-326, 1-327, 1-334, 1-352, 1-377, 1-395, 1-396, 1-406, 1-421, 1-422, 1-505, 1-507–1-513, 2-12, 2-13, 2-203, 2-222, 2-223, 2-230, 2-233–2-240, 2-246, 2-249, 2-272, 2-281, 2-283, 2-286, 2-293, 2-295, 2-296, 2-298, 2-299, 2-311, 2-313, 2-363, 2-365, 2-555, 3-54, 3-55, 3-127, 3-130, 3-137–3-140, 3-213, 3-215–3-218, 3-277, 3-315, 3-332, 3-387, 3-447, 3-474, 3-476, 3-625, 3-642, 3-662, 3-772, 3-792
benzothiadiazine, 3-644
benzylmorphine
    Peronine, 1-146
benzylpiperidines, 3-644
berberine, 1-147
Berger, Frank, 1-322, 2-10
Bergmann, Ernst von, 1-118
Bergson, Henri-Louis, 2-528
Beringer, K., 2-534

Berle, Milton, 2-222

Bernard, Claude, 1-190, 1-214, 1-234, 2-61, 2-259, 3-88, 3-106, 3-155

Bernheim, Hippolyte, 1-15

Bernthsen, August, 2-58

Bernthsen, Heinrich August, 2-125

Berrios, German F., 1-28, 3-326, 3-750

Bertan's polybromate elixir, 1-145

Berthe's Paste and Syrup, 1-127

Berthier Laboratories, 1-329

betel (Piper betle), 3-491

Bethe, Albrecht, 1-201

bhang, 2-482, *see* cannabis

Biedermann, Joseph, 3-245

bifeprunox, 3-649, 3-654

bile, 1-39–1-41, 1-43, 1-49, 1-127, 2-25, 2-330, 3-735, 3-738

bilirubin, 2-286

binding, 1-171, 1-174, 1-238, 1-242, 1-252, 1-255, 1-257, 1-259, 1-260, 1-262, 1-263, 1-265, 1-268, 1-281, 1-284, 1-369, 1-450, 1-484, 1-492, 1-493, 1-510, 2-85, 2-98, 2-148, 2-150, 2-152–2-154, 2-235, 2-236, 2-238, 2-239, 2-293, 2-386, 3-25, 3-52, 3-53, 3-65, 3-67, 3-193, 3-507, 3-508, 3-558, 3-560, 3-565, 3-566, 3-571, 3-583–3-587, 3-605, 3-634, 3-640, 3-663

binding sites, 1-284, 1-510, 2-234, 2-235, 2-238, 2-293, 2-420, 2-422, 3-656

Binding, Karl, 3-89

Bini, Lucio, 1-21, 2-337, 3-344, 3-346

Binswanger, Ludwig, 1-19, 1-20, *1-20*, 3-712

Binz, Karl, 1-110

biological theories, 1-xxvii, 1-206

biotransformation, 2-169, 2-283, 3-25

bipolar disorder, 1-245, 1-250, 1-267, 1-291, 1-296, 1-314, 1-335, 1-364, 1-379, 1-380, 1-445, 1-446, 2-7, 2-158, 2-189, 2-192, 2-193, 2-195–2-198, 2-203–2-211, 2-523, 3-52, 3-82, 3-181, 3-228, 3-245, 3-292, 3-293, 3-327, 3-334–3-336, 3-417, 3-474, 3-511, 3-512, 3-517, 3-520, 3-523, 3-524, 3-526, 3-527, 3-543, 3-582, 3-626, 3-650, 3-653, 3-654, 3-661

Birch, John, 2-335

bites, 1-460

bitter almonds, 1-119

bitter tincture, 1-138

bittersweet, 1-130

Bizzozero, Giulio, 1-191

black bang, *see* cannabis

black hellebore, *see* hellebore

Black, Joseph, 2-440

blackberries, 2-436

Bleckwenn, William J., 2-279

Bleuler, Eugen, *1-12*, 1-13, 2-276

Bleuler, Manfred, 1-xv, 1-18, 2-273, 2-534, 3-766

blindness, 2-431, 3-90, 3-202, 3-332, 3-344, 3-603

Bloch, C., 2-79

Bloch, Felix, 1-174, 1-442

blonanserin, 3-649

blood, 1-39, 1-40, 1-44, 1-48, 1-73, 1-88, 1-91, 1-118, 1-139, 1-141, 1-159, 1-184, 1-238, 1-240, 1-332, 1-359, 1-364, 1-375–1-381, 1-385, 1-441, 1-446, 1-449, 1-460, 1-466, 1-481, 1-490, 1-510, 2-7, 2-28, 2-33, 2-67, 2-79, 2-110, 2-171, 2-184, 2-195, 2-196, 2-254, 2-257, 2-285, 2-307, 2-309, 2-315, 2-330, 2-331, 2-354, 2-398, 2-442, 2-454, 2-490, 2-495, 2-497, 2-511, 2-514, 2-532, 3-22, 3-61, 3-66, 3-93,

3-132, 3-133, 3-173, 3-349,
3-375, 3-381, 3-467, 3-520,
3-526, 3-564, 3-570, 3-571,
3-603, 3-612, 3-652, 3-657,
3-740, 3-765, 3-787

blood-brain barrier, 1-305, 1-321, 1-341,
1-483, 2-191, 3-520, 3-612, 3-653

bloodletting, 1-xvii, 1-69, 2-325, 2-330,
2-331, 3-375, 3-380, 3-381, 3-739

bloodroot (Sanguinaria canadensis), 2-328

blue methylene, see methylene blue

Blue morning glory (Ipomoea indica),
3-797

Boccaccio, Giovanni, 2-436

Bocquillon-Limousin, Henri, 1-151

Boerhaave, Herman, 2-525

boldo, 1-139

boldo glycine, 1-146

bombesin, 3-600

Bonaparte, Marie, 3-503

bone, 1-329, 1-332, 1-442, 3-439, 3-568

bone marrow stimulants, 1-146

Bonhoeffer, Karl, 1-13

borderline personality disorder, 1-483,
2-160, 2-353, 3-217, 3-336,
3-523

Borelli, Giovanni Alfonso, 1-186

Borlase, John Bingham, 2-440

bornyval, 1-151

Bose, Kartick Chandra, 2-28, 2-453

Bouchardat, A., 1-123

Bouhler, Philip, 3-94, 3-100

Bovet, Daniel, 1-307, 2-56, 3-6

Bowlby, John, 3-415

Boyle, Robert, 2-439

bradycardia, 2-354

brain, 1-xiv, 1-xix, 1-xxiii, 1-xxvii, 1-9,
1-14, 1-27, 1-40, 1-43, 1-46,
1-48, 1-50, 1-53, 1-66, 1-70, 1-80, 1-93, 1-103, 1-105–1-107,

1-120, 1-127, 1-136, 1-147,
1-152, 1-154, 1-157, 1-161,
1-167, 1-168, 1-170–1-172,
1-174, 1-176, 1-184, 1-185,
1-191, 1-192, 1-199, 1-213–
1-229, 1-240, 1-241, 1-249,
1-253, 1-255, 1-259, 1-262,
1-265, 1-267–1-269, 1-277,
1-279, 1-284, 1-287, 1-292,
1-356–1-359, 1-364, 1-367–
1-369, 1-384, 1-407–1-409,
1-421, 1-422, 1-424, 1-441–
1-444, 1-446–1-452, 1-459,
1-462, 1-463, 1-465–1-472,
1-479–1-482, 1-485, 1-488,
1-490, 1-493, 1-506, 1-508–1-510, 1-514, 1-527, 1-528, 2-14,
2-15, 2-17, 2-38, 2-44, 2-85, 2-96, 2-106, 2-107, 2-111, 2-142,
2-144, 2-146, 2-150–2-154,
2-167, 2-191, 2-203, 2-222,
2-226, 2-235–2-237, 2-239,
2-247, 2-309, 2-310, 2-313,
2-325, 2-331, 2-332, 2-335,
2-337, 2-340–2-342, 2-347,
2-348, 2-357, 2-368, 2-386,
2-387, 2-390, 2-397, 2-398,
2-402, 2-408, 2-409, 2-420,
2-422, 2-461, 2-487, 2-495,
2-496, 2-510, 2-511, 3-5,
3-23, 3-78, 3-88, 3-99, 3-122,
3-206, 3-228, 3-238, 3-279–
3-281, 3-293, 3-298, 3-300,
3-322, 3-337, 3-344, 3-347,
3-348, 3-353, 3-355, 3-395,
3-399–3-401, 3-403, 3-404,
3-411, 3-414–3-418, 3-497,
3-504–3-510, 3-513, 3-514,
3-517, 3-520, 3-521, 3-525,
3-526, 3-545, 3-551–3-554,
3-558, 3-560, 3-562–3-566,
3-568, 3-570, 3-571, 3-582,
3-593–3-595, 3-598, 3-601,

3-604, 3-606, 3-610, 3-612,
3-631, 3-633, 3-639, 3-640,
3-644, 3-657, 3-662, 3-664,
3-668, 3-732, 3-735, 3-736,
3-738, 3-740, 3-766, 3-772,
3-797
brain damage, 1-176
brain diseases, 3-228, 3-560
brain lesion, 1-8
brain surgery, *see* lobotomy
Brain, Sir Russell, 3-15
Brandt, Karl, 3-94, 3-100
brandy, 2-329, 2-497, 2-498, 3-201
bretazenil, 3-663
Breuer, Josef, 1-15, 3-712
Brevital, *see* methohexital
Brill, Henry, 2-9, 2-42, 2-70
British Empire, 2-473, 3-190
Broadhurst, Alan, 3-9, 3-11
Broca, Paul, 1-118
Brodie, Bernard B., 1-465, 2-44, 2-131,
2-137, 3-765
bromal, 1-129, 1-146
bromaline, 1-146, 1-147
Bromameti iformina, 1-147
bromamide, 1-147
bromate, 1-127, 1-145
bromdiethylacetamide, 1-156
bromdiethylacetilurea, 1-156
bromide, 1-108, 1-109, 1-127, 1-129,
1-137–1-142, 1-144, 1-146–
1-148, 1-151, 1-152, 1-159,
1-160, 1-328, 1-352, 1-377,
2-4, 2-125, 2-220, 2-229,
2-258–2-261, 2-265–2-267,
2-272, 2-277, 2-306, 2-307,
2-329, 2-363, 2-512, 2-513,
2-522, 3-662, 3-771
bromidia, 1-140, 1-141, 1-147
brominated ethylene bromide, 1-147
bromocriptine, 1-492, 2-310, 3-771
Parlodel, 2-310
bromohemol, 1-149

bromperidol, 2-81
bromural, 1-156, 1-157, 1-160
bromvalerylurea, 1-156
bromvalidol, 1-151
valerianic ether of menthol, 1-151
bronchitis, 1-127
chronic, 2-519
bronchopneumonia, 2-274
Brooks, Charles, 2-277
Brouillet, André, *1-16*
Brown, John, 1-71, 2-518
Brown, Thomas, 1-101
Brown-Séquard, Charles Edouard,
2-259, 2-260, 2-519
Antineuralgic Pills, 2-519
brucine, 1-119
Bruno, E., 2-38
bryony (Bryonia dioica), 1-97
Buchheim, Rudolf, 1-110, 1-234, 2-256
bufotenine, 3-790
bulimia nervosa, 2-160, 2-161
Bumke, Oswald, 1-206, 3-747
Bunney, Jr., William, 2-137
Bunsen, Robert W., 2-267
buprenorphine, 2-308–2-310, 2-314, 2-
315, 2-510, 2-514, 3-54, 3-213,
3-645
Suboxone, 2-310
Subutex, 2-310
bupropion, 1-343, 2-351, 3-471, 3-644
Burckhardt, Gottlieb, 2-342
burns, 1-48, 1-121, 2-517, 3-251, 3-430,
3-437, 3-735
Burns, B. H., 2-132
Burton, Robert, 2-517, 2-521
buspirone, 1-326, 1-484, 2-245–2-247,
2-368, 2-370, 3-662, 3-664,
3-665
Bustamante, 3-801
butabarbital, 2-286, 3-140
butazone, 3-299
butethal, *see* butobarbital
butobarbital, 2-271, 2-272, 2-278

butethal, 2-271
Neonal, 1-160, 2-271
butorphanol, 2-420, 3-563
butyl/chloral, 1-148
butyl-chloral, 1-131, 1-132, 1-134, 1-146, 1-151
butyl-chloral hydrate, 1-160
butyrylcholinesterase (BuChE, BCHE), 2-315, 2-383
Byron, George, 2-439
BZD$_1$ receptor
agonist, 2-238, *see also* zolpidem

C

Cabaleiro, Manuel, 3-731, 3-748
Caballero, Juan Barcia, 3-721
Cabanis, Pierre Jean George, 3-187
cacao (Theobroma cacao), 1-346, 2-456
chocolate, 1-346, 2-110, 2-458, 2-494
seed, 2-456
Cactaceae, 2-464
Cade, John Frederick, 1-ix, 1-21, 1-154, 1-380, 1-418, 2-181, 3-14, 3-278, 3-504, 3-625
caffeine, 1-134, 1-143, 1-144, 1-153, 1-154, 1-160, 1-262, 1-346, 1-347, 2-6, 2-354, 2-451, 2-456, 2-496, 2-528, 2-531–2-533, 3-344, 3-350, 3-498, 3-660, 3-796
Cajal y Ramón, Santiago, 1-11, 1-168, 1-169, 1-190–1-199, 1-201–1-204, 1-206, 1-207, 1-234, 2-14, 2-487, 3-593, 3-711, 3-712, 3-714, 3-715, 3-722, 3-723, 3-730, 3-742, 3-743, 3-756, 3-757, 3-775
calabar bean (Physostigma venenosum), 1-130
Calamus (Acorus calamus), 2-463
calcium acetylhomotaurine, *see* acamprosate

calcium dobesilate, 3-299
calcium oxalate, 3-434
calcium tartrate, 1-152
Caldwell, Anne E., 1-xxiv, 1-xxv, 2-32
Calmeil, Louis Florentin, 1-105
calmodulin, 1-257, 1-260, 3-634
calyx, 1-199
Camellia sinensis, 1-346, 2-456
Cameron, D. Ewen, 2-276
cAMP, *see* cyclic adenosine monophosphate (cAMP)
Campderá, Francisco, 3-719
camphor, 1-90, 1-94, 1-97, 1-119, 1-127, 1-129, 1-137, 1-142, 1-146, 1-147, 1-150, 2-5, 2-325, 2-326, 2-329, 2-335, 2-336, 3-344
camphor bromide, 1-126, 1-127, 1-151
camphor laurel (Cinnamomum camphora), 2-329
camphora dye, 2-414
cancer, 1-121, 1-132, 1-291, 1-417, 2-40, 2-176, 2-398, 2-423, 2-447, 2-448, 2-521, 3-41, 3-52, 3-293, 3-306, 3-448, 3-457, 3-467, 3-472–3-476, 3-570, 3-646
candahol, 1-147
cannabichromene, 2-520
cannabicyclol, 2-520
delta-8-THC, 2-520
cannabidiol, 1-304, 2-520, 2-523
cannabigerol, 2-520
cannabina, 1-146
cannabina tannate, 1-151
cannabinoid, 1-237, 1-243, 1-406, 2-447, 2-461, 2-521, 3-660
cannabinol, 1-155, 1-158, 1-304, 2-519
cannabinone, 1-148
cannabis, 1-151, 1-159, 1-303, 1-304, 2-6, 2-265, 2-329, 2-415, 2-432, 2-434, 2-447, 2-449, 2-451, 2-460, 2-461, 2-471, 2-472, 2-482–2-484, 2-505, 2-515–2-523, 3-54, 3-189,

3-197, 3-205, 3-211, 3-432, 3-433, 3-439, 3-491, 3-494, 3-496, 3-497, 3-660

Cannabis indica, 2-3, 2-305, 2-306, 2-329, 2-518

Cannabis sativa, 1-148, 2-361, 2-518

African, 2-487

bang, 3-432, 3-439

bangue, 2-517

black bang, 3-439

dawamesk, 2-518

dawamsec, 2-5, 2-6

decriminalization, 2-419

effects on intraocular pressure, 2-520

extract, 2-518, 3-197

hashish, 1-xxiv, 1-106, 1-124, 1-131, 1-132, 1-155, 1-162, 2-5, 2-432, 2-436, 2-439, 2-449, 2-460, 2-515, 2-517, 2-518, 2-521, 2-522, 3-185, 3-197, 3-492, 3-495–3-497

hemp, 1-xxiii, 1-140, 1-155, 2-361, 2-461, 2-515, 2-517, 3-197, 3-432

Indian hemp, 1-131, 1-132, 1-146, 1-147, 1-155, 2-3, 2-518

pollen, 3-432

red bang, 3-439

white bang, 3-439

cannabis consumption by the very same, 2-484

cannabis receptor CB-1, 3-660

cannabitriol, 2-520

CBT, 2-313, 3-401

Cannon, Walter Bradford, 1-154, 2-397

capacitation, 3-137

Capgras, Joseph, 1-12

capillary electrophoresis (CE), 1-359, 1-363, 1-365, 1-367, 1-382, 2-491, 3-51

Capone, Alphonse, 3-203

captodiame
captodiamine, 2-82, 3-763

captodiamine, *see* captodiame

captopril, 3-307

carbamazepine, 1-334, 1-364, 1-379, 1-451, 2-189, **2-193**, 2-193–2-197, 2-203, 2-204, 2-206, 2-208, 2-209, 2-211, 2-278, 2-313, 2-367, 3-514, 3-517
Tegretol, 2-313

carbomal, 1-160

carbon dioxide, 1-160, 2-285, 2-442, 3-384

carbon monoxide poisoning, 3-94

carbonate, 1-152, 3-278

carbonic anhydrase, 1-335, 2-208, 2-210, 3-562

carcinoma, 3-457

cardiac medicines, 1-130

cardiac muscle, 1-234

cardiasthenic, 1-144

Cardiazol, *see* pentylenetetrazol

cardiazol therapy, 2-272

cardiovascular disease, 1-291

cardol, 1-148

Cardozo, Benjamin, 3-169

cariprazine, 3-651
RGH-188, 3-651

carisoprodol, 1-322
Soma, 1-195, 1-199, 1-202, 1-322, 2-464, 2-482, 3-315, 3-430, 3-552

carotene, 3-364

carotid artery, 2-286

Carraz, George, 2-190

Carrión, Esteban, 2-443

cartilage, 1-187, 2-7

carvacrol, 1-146

Casaña, Julian, 1-123

Casmann, Otto, 1-58

cast, 3-246

Castel, Robert, 1-23

Castellanos, Gastón, 3-801

castor, 1-119, 1-129, 1-146, 1-151, 2-5

castoreum, 1-73

castorine, 1-119

catabolism, 1-336, 1-339, 3-645

Catapres, *see* clonidine

cataract, 1-122, 2-441

catatonia, 1-xxv, 2-279, 2-402, 3-790

catecholamines, 1-240, 1-254, 1-283, 1-304, 1-336, 1-462, 1-466–1-468, 1-471, 1-480, 2-15, 2-16, 2-40, 2-107, 2-110, 2-144, 2-152, 2-158, 3-635, 3-646, 3-771

Catha edulis, *see* khat

cathinone, 3-796

Cavendish, Henry, 2-440

Caventou, Joseph Bienaimé, 1-110, 1-118

CBT, *see* cannabitriol

CCK-A receptor, 3-659

CCK-B receptor, 3-659, 3-666

CDER, *see* Center for Drug Evaluation and Research (CDER)

cDNA, *see* complementary DNA (cDNA)

Celastrus edulis, 1-133

celecoxib, 3-646, 3-661

celery, 1-119

cell, 1-168, 1-172, 1-174, 1-186–1-191, 1-193, 1-195–1-197, 1-199, 1-201–1-203, 1-206, 1-226, 1-229, 1-234, 1-250, 1-252, 1-253, 1-257, 1-259, 1-260, 1-262–1-265, 1-269, 1-278, 1-279, 1-283, 1-287, 1-482, 1-483, 1-528, 1-530, 2-144, 2-390, 3-5, 3-61, 3-66, 3-280, 3-399, 3-514, 3-517, 3-526, 3-546, 3-550, 3-552–3-554, 3-556, 3-558, 3-560, 3-562, 3-564, 3-565, 3-567–3-571, 3-600, 3-643, 3-645, 3-662

cell division, 1-188, 1-257

Center for Drug Evaluation and Research (CDER), 3-51, 3-53

Central Intelligence Agency (CIA), 2-276, 2-537, 2-549, 3-237, 3-496

central nervous system (CNS), 1-xxviii, 1-74, 1-75, 1-134, 1-154, 1-155, 1-159, 1-168, 1-170, 1-172, 1-174, 1-202, 1-205, 1-215–1-219, 1-233, 1-236, 1-238, 1-240–1-243, 1-250, 1-253, 1-254, 1-257, 1-260, 1-263–1-265, 1-267, 1-303, 1-305, 1-319, 1-322, 1-324, 1-328, 1-329, 1-333, 1-335, 1-345, 1-346, 1-350, 1-406, 1-407, 1-409, 1-415, 1-420, 1-481, 1-482, 1-487, 1-488, 1-490, 1-492, 1-493, 2-32, 2-45, 2-94, 2-95, 2-111, 2-141, 2-206, 2-219, 2-220, 2-225, 2-235, 2-238, 2-254, 2-285, 2-286, 2-294, 2-347–2-350, 2-354, 2-355, 2-357, 2-361, 2-386, 2-397, 2-398, 2-404, 2-408, 2-420, 2-422, 2-453, 2-454, 2-527, 2-529, 2-557, 3-15, 3-207, 3-214, 3-215, 3-281, 3-291, 3-330, 3-348, 3-349, 3-361, 3-411, 3-509, 3-510, 3-518, 3-548, 3-550, 3-558, 3-560, 3-568, 3-585, 3-587, 3-594–3-596, 3-598–3-603, 3-606, 3-607, 3-609, 3-628, 3-640, 3-657, 3-660, 3-662, 3-666, 3-769, 3-795–3-797

central nervous system stimulants, 1-160

cerebellum, 1-190, 1-195, 1-196, 1-201, 1-204, 2-422, 3-598

cerebral hemorrhage, 2-59, 2-286

cerebral sedative, 1-147

cerebral trauma, 2-524

cerebrospinal fluid, 1-369, 1-443, 1-472,

1-481, 2-96, 3-559, 3-561, 3-640

cerebrum, 1-143

Cerf, Vinton G., 3-616

cerium, 1-147

Cerletti, Ugo, 1-xxiv, 1-21, 2-337, 2-338, 2-407, 3-344, 3-346, 3-347, 3-358, 3-714

Cervello, Vincenzo, 2-267

Cervina Fumouze, 1-143

Cesamet, *see* nabilone

CGS-19755, *see* Selfotel (CGS-19755)

Chambers, W.W., 1-174

Charaka (Charka), 2-26, 2-27, 3-125

Charaka Samhita, 2-26, 2-27, 3-125

Charcot, Jean-Martin, *1-16*

Charcot, Jean-Martin, 1-14, 3-344, 3-711

Charles University, 2-168

Charpentier, Paul, 1-308, 1-358, 1-420, 2-7, 2-58, 2-60, 2-229, 3-6, 3-361, 3-475

Chaslin, Philippe, 3-729

chavicol, 3-796

chelerythrine, 3-661

chelidonine, 1-155

Chen Shih-Kung, 3-125

Chen, Graham, 3-22

Chiang Kai-shek, 2-508

Chiarugi, Vincenzo, 1-3, 1-84

chicory, 1-90

Ching, Shen-Nung Pen-tsao, 3-432

chiral , 1-359, 1-361, 1-363

chloral, 1-109, 1-111, 1-118, 1-127, 1-131, 1-132, 1-134, 1-135, 1-137, 1-139, 1-140, 1-144, 1-148–1-151, 1-158, 1-160, 1-305, 2-257, 2-293, 2-307, 2-329, 2-512

chloral amylene, *see* dormiol

chloral hydrate, 1-110, 1-140, 1-142, 1-147, 1-157–1-159, 1-305, 2-4, 2-220, 2-229, 2-254–2-258,

2-265, 2-266, 2-276, 2-305, 2-306, 2-363, 2-445, 2-513, 2-520, 2-522, 2-555, 3-491, 3-496

chloralose, 1-148

chloramphenicol, 3-299

chlordiazepoxide, 1-ix, 1-xxiv, 1-323, 1-352, 1-397, 1-421, 1-422, 1-506, 2-13, 2-230–2-232, 2-283, 2-311, 2-366, 2-408, 2-555, 2-560, 3-217, 3-277, 3-504, 3-755, 3-772, 3-792

Librium, 1-323, 1-506, 2-232, 2-311

methaminodiazepoxide, 2-231, 2-366

RO 5-0690, 2-231

chloretone, *see* chlorobutanol

chloric ether, 2-330

chlorimipramine, *see* clomipramine

chlorobutanol, 1-160

chloretone, 1-148

chlorodyne, 2-519

chloroform, 1-106, 1-108, 1-111, 1-118, 1-119, 1-129, 1-131, 1-132, 1-140, 1-146, 1-148, 1-149, 1-151, 1-305, 1-416, 2-253, 2-254, 2-256, 2-257, 2-266, 2-444, 2-446, 2-448, 2-449, 2-505

chloroformed acetone, 1-147

chlorosis, 1-137, 1-143, 1-148, 1-149

chlorphenamine, 1-307

chlorpromazine
    discovery of, 3-361

chlorpromazine (CPZ), 1-ix, 1-xxvii, 1-21, 1-22, 1-117, 1-154, 1-162, 1-167, 1-170, 1-277, 1-307–1-309, 1-311, 1-316, 1-319, 1-322, 1-323, 1-334, 1-336, 1-358, 1-383, 1-384, 1-420, 1-421, 1-459, 1-460, 1-468, 1-470, 1-479, 2-7–2-10, 2-12, 2-13, 2-16, 2-17, 2-23,

2-24, 2-27, 2-32–2-35, 2-37, 2-38, 2-41, 2-42, 2-45, 2-55, 2-60–2-63, 2-65–2-71, 2-75, 2-77, 2-80, 2-82, 2-85, 2-88, 2-94–2-96, 2-126, 2-127, 2-133, 2-184, 2-186, 2-187, 2-189, 2-194, 2-219, 2-222, 2-223, 2-225, 2-229, 2-230, 2-283, 2-343, 2-365, 2-406, 2-407, 2-555, 3-3, 3-5–3-8, 3-10, 3-11, 3-15, 3-16, 3-35, 3-122, 3-133, 3-277–3-279, 3-282, 3-361–3-365, 3-368, 3-369, 3-472, 3-475, 3-476, 3-504, 3-594, 3-755, 3-761–3-763, 3-766, 3-770, 3-773

Largactil, 1-162, 1-479, 2-62, 2-68, 2-69, 3-8, 3-762

Orthotimic, 3-766

Thorazine, 1-527, 2-69, 2-70, 2-130, 3-8

chlorprothixene, 1-311, 2-75, 2-85, 2-86

CHMP, *see* Committee for Medicinal Products for Human Use (CHMP)

chocolate, *see* cacao (Theobroma cacao)

cholera, 1-121, 2-10, 2-27, 2-448

cholestasis, 3-467

cholinergic, 1-205, 1-242, 1-337, 1-341, 1-343, 1-397, 2-99, 2-234, 2-382, 2-386, 2-388, 2-390, 2-391, 2-510, 3-218, 3-453, 3-457, 3-510, 3-561, 3-596, 3-647, 3-654, 3-769

Chopra, Ram Nath, 2-29

chorea, 1-121, 1-127, 1-131, 1-132, 1-136, 1-141, 1-142, 1-149, 1-157–1-159, 2-447, 2-448, 3-90, 3-476

choroid plexus, 2-150

Christianity, 2-434, 2-448, 2-464, 2-473, 3-294, 3-706

Christie, Agatha, 3-493, 3-496–3-499

chromatin, 3-565, 3-566

chromosomes, 1-190, 1-291, 3-506, 3-544

chronoamperometry, 1-367, 1-368

Churchill, Winston, 3-8

CI-400, *see* eticyclidine

CIA, *see* Central Intelligence Agency (CIA)

Cicero, Marco Tulio, 1-167

cimetidine, 2-558, 3-464–3-466

Cimicifuga, 1-147

cinchona, 1-72, 3-374

cinnabar, 1-65

cinnamic acid, 3-796

Cinnamomum camphora, *see* camphor laurel (Cinnamomum camphora)

cinnamon, 1-68, 1-138, 2-414, 2-452, 2-518

cinnarizine, 3-467

CINP, *see* Collegium Internationale Neuro-Psychopharmacologicum (CINP)

Circaea, 2-432

cirrhosis, 2-313, 2-498

cisplatin, 3-473

citalopram, 1-341, 1-343, 1-352, 1-356, 1-360, 1-362, 1-484, 2-141, 2-148, 2-157, 2-168, 2-174, 2-175, 3-456, 3-642

citrofen, 1-146, 1-147

CL 284,846, *see* zaleplon

Clérambault, Gatian de, *1-12*, 1-13, 1-18

CL-218,872, *see* zolpidem

Clark, A. J., 1-171

Clarke, William, 2-443

Claude, Pierre Jean, 1-74

Cleghorn, Robert A., 2-398

Clin, 1-127

clinical trial, 1-xxvii, 1-357, 1-363, 1-376, 1-383, 1-415–1-424, 1-427, 1-429, 1-431, 1-434,

1-460, 2-7, 2-8, 2-29, 2-32,
2-35, 2-79, 2-85, 2-94, 2-95,
2-108, 2-110, 2-142, 2-156,
2-159, 2-168, 2-174, 2-186,
2-187, 2-197, 2-204, 2-205,
2-207, 2-210, 2-230, 2-232,
2-240, 2-294, 2-314, 2-371,
2-388, 2-390, 2-391, 2-548,
2-549, 3-11–3-14, 3-21, 3-25,
3-37, 3-42, 3-49, 3-55, 3-61,
3-65, 3-67, 3-81, 3-82, 3-87,
3-105–3-107, 3-112–3-114,
3-131, 3-132, 3-156, 3-157,
3-163, 3-165, 3-176, 3-180,
3-239, 3-242, 3-252, 3-255,
3-305–3-308, 3-315, 3-362,
3-364, 3-367, 3-368, 3-385,
3-389, 3-462, 3-641, 3-644,
3-646, 3-647, 3-652, 3-653,
3-655, 3-660, 3-794, 3-798
Cloëtta, Max, 2-272
clobenzorex, 3-67, 3-68
clomipramine, 1-336, 1-357, 1-484,
2-113, 2-133, 2-135, 2-137,
2-142, 2-148, 2-156, 2-168,
2-171, 2-172, 2-174, 2-175,
3-3, 3-12, 3-13, 3-15, 3-16,
3-144, 3-455, 3-747
Anafranil, 2-133
chlorimipramine, 3-12
monochlorimipramine, 2-133
clonazepam, 1-334, 1-378, 2-196, 2-559,
3-217, 3-476
clone, 1-278, 1-280, 1-283–1-285, 3-600
clonidine, 1-327, 1-489, 2-309, 2-314, 3-
331, 3-460
Catapres, 2-309
cloning, 1-xxv, 1-171, 1-254, 1-280,
1-281, 1-283–1-286, 1-288–
1-290, 2-421, 2-425, 3-543,
3-545, 3-662
clorazepate, 1-507
Tranxene, 1-507

clorgiline, 3-642
clorgyline, 2-111, 2-112, 3-767
clorgyline, see clorgiline
clorotepine, 3-653
Clostridium acetobutylicum, 2-271
Clouston, Thomas, 2-522
clover, 2-414
clozapine, 1-238, 1-294, 1-295, 1-311,
1-312, 1-358, 1-361, 1-471,
1-472, 2-86, 2-93, 2-95–
2-100, 2-366, 3-58, 3-61,
3-132–3-135, 3-287, 3-298,
3-299, 3-308, 3-310, 3-316,
3-473–3-475, 3-506, 3-508,
3-567, 3-582, 3-648–3-650,
3-652–3-655, 3-658, 3-659,
3-661, 3-773
Clozaril, 3-133
receptor, 3-650
Clozaril, see clozapine
CME, see continuing medical education
(CME)
coca, 1-xxiii, 1-119, 1-127, 1-134, 1-140,
1-151, 1-303, 1-356, 1-528,
1-529, 2-305, 2-348, 2-445,
2-446, 2-455, **2-476**, 2-476–
2-478, 2-525–2-530, 3-198,
3-209, 3-497
coca leaves, 1-529, 2-348, 2-455, 2-
471, 2-525, 2-528
drink, 2-478
Erythroxylon, 2-525
Erythroxylon coca, 2-445, 2-455
Erythroxylum coca, 1-529, 2-476,
3-197
French Wine Cocaine, 2-528
leaves, 2-477, 2-478, 3-197, 3-210
tea, 2-478
Vin Mariani, 2-455, 2-478, 2-527, 2-
528, 3-198
Coca-Cola
decocainized, 2-478
cocaine, 1-xxiv, 1-112, 1-119, 1-129,

1-134, 1-137, 1-146, 1-151, 1-159, 1-233, 1-240, 1-241, 1-304, 1-352, 1-395, 1-405, 1-408, 1-469, 1-470, 1-529, 1-530, 2-5, 2-32, 2-44, 2-305, 2-306, 2-310, 2-311, 2-314–2-316, 2-347–2-349, 2-445, 2-446, 2-451, 2-455, 2-456, 2-471, **2-476**, 2-477, 2-478, 2-487, 2-494, 2-505, 2-523, 2-524, 2-526–2-531, 2-562, 3-54, 3-189, 3-197–3-199, 3-201, 3-205, 3-209–3-211, 3-316, 3-491, 3-497, 3-498, 3-504, 3-563, 3-564, 3-566, 3-762, 3-765

cocaine vaccine, 2-314

dependence, 2-310, 2-311, 2-314, 3-198

cocoa, *see* cacao (Theobroma cacao)

Cocteau, Jean, 3-492

cod liver oil, 1-152, 3-4

codeine, 1-119, 1-121, 1-127, 1-131, 1-151, 1-156, 2-305, 2-306, 2-416, 2-453, 2-505, 3-54, 3-189

codon, 3-512, 3-569

cognitive disorder, 1-530, 2-381–2-383, 2-386, 2-387, 2-391, 3-653

Cohen, N., 2-398

colchicine, 1-130, 1-151

Coleridge, Samuel Taylor, 2-439, 2-440, 3-492

colic, 1-121, 2-448, 2-511, 2-525

Collard, J., 2-79

collateral, 1-196

Collegium Internationale Neuro-Psychopharmacologicum (CINP), 1-xxviii, 2-8, 2-9, 2-129, 2-168, 2-294, 3-35, 3-761, 3-768, 3-794

colocynth, 1-42

Colombier, Jean, 1-81–1-83

colubrine, 1-119

coma, 1-120, 1-124, 1-139, 2-59, 2-113, 2-285, 2-339, 2-340, 2-405, 2-448, 3-740

comacum, 2-463

combinatorial chemistry, 1-351, 3-755

Committee for Medicinal Products for Human Use (CHMP), 3-51, 3-52

common cold, 1-417, 3-245

common sundew, 1-146

complementary DNA (cDNA), 1-171, 1-278, 1-281, 1-283, 1-284, 1-286, 2-235, 3-526, 3-527, 3-546–3-548, 3-551, 3-568

compliance, 1-377, 1-383, 2-168, 2-175, 2-314, 3-107, 3-121, 3-131, 3-132, 3-179, 3-314

computed tomography (CT), 1-174, 1-441, 1-442, 3-349, 3-358

Concordin, *see* protriptyline

Condrau, G., 2-535

conduct disorder, 3-244, 3-402

cone, 3-187, 3-562

confusion, 1-25, 1-38, 1-75, 1-119, 1-160, 1-430, 2-65, 2-67, 2-197, 3-64, 3-234, 3-249, 3-349, 3-408, 3-745

congenital, 3-49, 3-90, 3-188, 3-607

Congress of Medical Supporters of Wine, 2-494

connective tissue, 1-229

Conolly, John, 1-99

Conti, Leonardo, 3-93, 3-100

continuing medical education (CME), 3-38, 3-40, 3-41, 3-240, 3-242, 3-253

contraceptives, 2-209, 2-558

Contralin, *see* disulfiram

convalescence, 1-91, 1-93, 1-94, 1-144, 2-42, 2-496

Convolvulaceae, *see* Morning glory (Convolvulaceae)

Index

Convulex, *see* valproic acid
convulsions, 1-62, 1-127, 1-131, 1-136,
        1-139–1-142, 1-144, 1-145,
        1-506,   2-5,   2-191,   2-221,
        2-277, 2-286, 2-306, 2-328,
        2-333, 2-336, 2-337, 2-339,
        2-352, 2-435, 2-448, 2-514,
        2-532,   3-22,   3-67,   3-215,
        3-344–3-347, 3-349, 3-352,
        3-604, 3-656, 3-658
Cooper, David, 1-22
Coppen, Alec, 2-137
copper, 1-73, 1-127, 3-620
coramine, *see* nikethamide
cordol, 1-146
Corkwood (Duboisia mioporcides),
        1-130, 1-155
cornea, 1-193
cortex, 1-139, 1-154, 1-156, 1-174,
        1-183, 1-191, 1-196, 1-213,
        1-214, 1-216, 1-218, 1-220,
        1-223–1-225, 1-227, 1-292,
        1-295, 1-444, 1-448, 1-491,
        1-493, 1-530, 1-531, 2-14,
        2-15,   2-147, 2-151, 2-152,
        2-158, 2-342, 2-386, 3-399,
        3-401, 3-507, 3-509, 3-517,
        3-520, 3-521, 3-527, 3-562,
        3-563, 3-596, 3-598, 3-601,
        3-606, 3-609, 3-630, 3-634,
        3-636, 3-645, 3-646, 3-648,
        3-652, 3-653, 3-662, 3-773
corticosteroids, 2-399, 3-640
corticotropin, *see* adrenocorticotropic
        hormone (ACTH)
cortisol, *see* hydrocortisone
cough, 1-108, 1-127, 1-131, 1-142,
        1-156, 2-285, 2-510, 2-511,
        2-519, 3-189
    convulsive, 1-121
    medicine, 2-510
Coulter, John, 2-534
coumarin, 1-129, 1-329

CP-101,606, *see* traxoprodil
cranial, 1-132, 3-88, 3-187
cranium, 2-335, 3-187
criminology, 1-7, 3-186–3-188, 3-499
crocodile dung, 3-375
Cromwell, Oliver, 3-380
Crusades, 2-472
crystallized aconite, *see* aconitine
CT, *see* computed tomography (CT)
Cuenca, Eduardo, 1-xxviii, 3-459, 3-761,
        3-765, 3-767
Cullen, William, 2-441, 3-741
curare, 1-130, 1-133, 1-134, 1-234, 2-61,
        2-71, 2-338, 2-447, 3-349
Cushing syndrome, 2-399
CX-516, 3-644, 3-658
    Ampalex, 3-658
cyanosis, 1-136, 2-275
cyclic   adenosine   monophosphate
        (cAMP), 1-255, 1-257, 1-264,
        1-265, 1-267, 2-152, 2-153,
        2-408, 2-534, 3-94, 3-513,
        3-598, 3-600, 3-606, 3-610,
        3-630, 3-631, 3-633–3-635,
        3-637, 3-792
cyclic imide, 1-333
cyclooxygenase-2 inhibitors, 3-661
cyclothiazide, 3-644
Cymbalta, *see* duloxetine
cyproheptadine, 3-467
cystic fibrosis, 3-543, 3-568
cytochrome, 1-265, 1-267, 1-294, 1-383,
        2-169, 2-170, 2-229, 2-285, 3-
        567, 3-584, 3-585
cytomegalovirus retinitis, 3-568
cytoplasm, 1-263, 3-518, 3-552, 3-570
cytoskeleton, 1-260

D

d'Abano, Pietro, 3-380
Dörner, Klaus, 1-23, 1-102, 1-104
d-tubocurarine, *see* tubocurarine

4-25

Dale, Henry Halett, 1-153, 1-169, 1-235, 2-3, 2-14, 3-5, 3-6

Dale, Henry Hallett, 1-205, 1-235, 3-593

Dalmane, *see* flurazepam

Daquin, Joseph, 1-3, 1-61, 1-75, 1-83

DAR-0100, *see* dihydrexidine

Darwin, Charles R., 1-9, 3-411

Datura, 1-106, 1-119, 1-130, 2-3, 2-265, 2-361, 2-439, 2-445, 2-448, 2-517

    Datura suaveolens, 3-797

daturine, *see* hyoscyamine

Daumezon, Georges, 2-56–2-58, 2-81

Davies, D.L., 2-35

Davy, Humphry, 2-440

dawamesk, *see* cannabis

dawamsec, *see* cannabis

de Boor, Wolfgang, 1-xxv

de Cárdenas, Juan, 2-498

de Castro, Velázquez, 1-135

de Chauliac, Guy, 2-436, 2-506

de Goya, Francisco, 2-435, 2-439

de Heredia, Pedro Miguel, 3-735, 3-739

de la Fuente Muñiz, Ramón, 3-801

de León, Pedro Ponce, 3-710

de Luzuriaga, Ignacio María, 3-741

de Maeztu, Ramiro, 3-730

de Mallorca, Palma, 3-707

de Mondeville, Henri, 2-431

de Nantes Barrera, Oliva Sabuco, 3-708, 3-735

de Quincey, Thomas, 2-509

de Sahagún, Bernardino, 2-534

de San Juan, Juan Huarte, 1-46, 3-707, 3-735, 3-736

de Santa Cruz, Alfonso Ponce, 3-735, 3-738

de Ulloa, Antonio, 2-525

de Unamuno, Miguel, 3-730

de Zárate, Agustin, 3-497

Deadly Nightshade, *see* Belladonna (Atropa belladonna)

deafness, 2-511, 3-90

deamination, 2-12, 2-106, 3-511

death, 1-52, 1-80, 1-93, 1-117, 1-120, 1-121, 1-124, 1-132, 1-139, 1-260, 1-265, 1-407, 2-29, 2-40, 2-56, 2-61, 2-113, 2-220, 2-281, 2-282, 2-310, 2-332, 2-335, 2-337, 2-340, 2-343, 2-360, 2-387, 2-389, 2-434, 2-435, 2-437, 2-448, 2-475, 2-477, 2-515, 2-551, 3-22, 3-24, 3-81, 3-97, 3-99, 3-100, 3-109, 3-110, 3-188, 3-218, 3-235, 3-237, 3-257, 3-284, 3-291, 3-322, 3-328, 3-345–3-347, 3-375, 3-389, 3-430, 3-434, 3-492, 3-496, 3-498, 3-499, 3-563, 3-603, 3-612, 3-667, 3-669, 3-710, 3-715, 3-722, 3-738–3-740, 3-788, 3-790

    sudden, 3-68, 3-198, 3-472

decarboxylation, 2-106

Declaration of Hawaii, 3-78, 3-108, 3-109, 3-127

Declaration of Helsinki, 3-90, 3-101, 3-104–3-108, 3-127, 3-154, 3-156, 3-161, 3-252, 3-389

Declaration of Human Rights, 3-153, 3-258

Declaration of Madrid, 1-xxvii, 3-109, 3-110, 3-127, 3-137, 3-158

degeneration theory, 1-7–1-10, 1-107

dehydration, 2-517, 3-416

dehydrobenzperidol, *see* droperidol

Dejerine, Jules, 1-14

del Campo, Luis Vela, 3-347

del Pino, Carlos Castilla, 3-716, 3-723, 3-731, 3-749

Delabarre, Edmund Burke, 2-522

Delalande Research, 1-341

Delay, Jean, 1-ix, 1-xxv, 1-21, 1-167, 1-309, 2-34, 2-65, 2-67, 2-75, 2-126, 2-184, 2-365, 2-537, 2-549, 3-6, 3-122, 3-363,

3-504, 3-594, 3-790
Delgado, Honorio, 3-745, 3-802
delirious rage, 1-131
delirium, 1-6, 1-12, 1-18–1-21, 1-86,
 1-90, 1-131, 1-140, 1-144, 2-5,
 2-267, 2-273, 2-329, 2-332,
 2-355, 2-485, 2-513, 3-346,
 3-475, 3-499, 3-739, 3-745,
 3-749
 alcoholic, 1-131
 chronic, 1-5, 1-6, 1-12
 delirium tremens, 1-108, 1-121,
  1-127, 1-131, 1-132, 1-134,
  1-142, 1-157, 1-158, 2-35,
  2-79, 2-274, 2-339, 2-447,
  2-496–2-498, 2-513, 3-494
 febrile, 1-65, 1-131, 1-157
 manic, 1-131
 nervous, 1-121
 schizophrenic, 3-723
 Solenaceae induced, 1-124
 systematic, 1-11
 terminal, 1-15
 with mania, 1-5
delphine, see delphinine
delphinine
 delphine, 1-146
delta sleep inducing peptide, 1-222
delta-8-THC, see cannabicyclol
delta-9-THC, see tetrahydrocannabinol
 (THC)
Delysid, see lysergic acid diethylamide
 (LSD)
dementia, 1-5, 1-11, 1-18, 1-19, 1-43,
 1-65, 1-105, 1-108, 1-143,
 1-449, 2-5, 2-353, 2-381, 2-
 386, 2-387, 2-533, 3-80, 3-83,
 3-128, 3-174, 3-176, 3-187,
 3-234, 3-293, 3-447, 3-462,
 3-545, 3-559, 3-561, 3-603,
 3-721, 3-736, 3-741, 3-775
 Alzheimer's Disease, 2-366
 boxer's, 3-604

 cerebrovascular, 2-381
 epileptic, 1-107
 hypochondriac, 1-107
 hysterical, 1-107, 1-142
 paralytic, 1-105, 2-229, 2-338,
  2-339
 precocious dementia, 1-11–1-13
 senile, 3-476, 3-795
dementia praecox, 1-18, 2-181, 2-229, 3-
 89
dendrite, 1-203, 1-263
Deniker, Pierre, 1-ix, 1-21, 1-167, 1-309,
 1-420, 1-421, 1-460, 2-8,
 2-10, 2-34, 2-35, 2-37, 2-38,
 2-65–2-67, 2-69, 2-71, 2-75,
 2-81, 2-86, 2-93–2-95, 2-99,
 2-126, 2-184, 2-365, 2-407,
 3-6, 3-122, 3-363, 3-364,
 3-504, 3-790
deoxyribonucleic acid (DNA), 1-179,
 1-226, 1-229, 1-243, 1-252,
 1-268, 1-278–1-283, 1-289,
 1-295, 1-340, 1-384, 2-421,
 3-526, 3-544, 3-546–3-548,
 3-550, 3-551, 3-553, 3-554,
 3-560, 3-565–3-570, 3-610
Depakene, see valproate
Depakine, see valproate
Depakote, see valproate
Depakote Sprinkle, see valproic acid
Depamide, see valpromide
depolarization, 1-260, 2-386
deprenyl, see selegiline
depressant, 1-146, 1-308, 1-311, 1-316,
 1-324, 1-326, 1-328, 1-329,
 1-420, 1-460, 2-11, 2-230,
 2-254, 2-258, 2-285, 2-286,
 3-25, 3-54, 3-214, 3-215, 3-664
depression, 1-ix, 1-xxiv, 1-70, 1-133,
 1-140, 1-142, 1-144, 1-151,
 1-152, 1-162, 1-176–1-178,
 1-262, 1-314, 1-326, 1-337,
 1-340, 1-341, 1-345, 1-349,

1-351, 1-356–1-358, 1-370, 1-397, 1-399, 1-418, 1-420, 1-421, 1-429, 1-436, 1-449, 1-471, 1-479–1-496, 1-513, 2-4, 2-5, 2-7, 2-12, 2-13, 2-15, 2-16, 2-29, 2-40, 2-41, 2-44, 2-45, 2-67, 2-94, 2-105–2-112, 2-115, 2-125, 2-126, 2-128, 2-129, 2-131, 2-132, 2-135–2-137, 2-141, 2-142, 2-153, 2-154, 2-156–2-161, 2-167, 2-168, 2-171, 2-176, 2-177, 2-186, 2-191, 2-204, 2-205, 2-211, 2-220, 2-246, 2-247, 2-285, 2-310, 2-311, 2-327, 2-336, 2-347, 2-348, 2-350, 2-357, 2-361, 2-370, 2-399, 2-401, 2-402, 2-404, 2-407, 2-408, 2-448, 2-458, 2-459, 2-513–2-515, 2-519, 2-522–2-525, 2-527, 2-530, 2-531, 2-538, 2-557, 3-5, 3-11, 3-22, 3-52, 3-64, 3-65, 3-67, 3-82, 3-84, 3-132, 3-174, 3-179, 3-187, 3-216, 3-227, 3-245, 3-250, 3-277, 3-278, 3-280, 3-282, 3-284, 3-285, 3-292, 3-306, 3-310, 3-312, 3-313, 3-315, 3-316, 3-321, 3-331, 3-332, 3-343, 3-351, 3-352, 3-354, 3-365–3-367, 3-386, 3-387, 3-389, 3-401, 3-415, 3-417, 3-419, 3-420, 3-438, 3-450, 3-452, 3-453, 3-455–3-457, 3-459, 3-468, 3-471, 3-474, 3-510, 3-511, 3-513, 3-518, 3-520, 3-522–3-524, 3-552, 3-562, 3-582, 3-587, 3-611, 3-626, 3-628–3-631, 3-633, 3-635, 3-636, 3-638–3-642, 3-644–3-648, 3-654, 3-668, 3-669, 3-738, 3-770, 3-790, 3-793, 3-794

depressive disorder, 2-33, 2-69, 3-292, 3-325, 3-331, 3-524, 3-646
  major, 2-158, 2-171, 2-172, 3-228, 3-511, 3-518, 3-520, 3-521, 3-523, 3-527, 3-562
dermatitis, 2-259
  atopic, 3-466
Derosne, Charles Louis, 1-110
Descartes, René, 1-184, 1-213, 3-395, 3-741
deserpidine, 2-10
desipramine, 1-336, 1-337, 1-357, 1-361, 1-383, 1-490, 2-16, 2-132, 2-142, 2-144, 2-146, 2-156, 2-159, 2-168, 2-191, 3-12, 3-451–3-453, 3-517, 3-633, 3-634, 3-642, 3-772
  desmethylimipramine, 3-634, 3-765
  DMI, 3-634, 3-645, 3-765
desmethylimipramine, see desipramine
dewtry, see Datura
Dexamyl, 2-282
dexfenfluramine, 2-350, **3-67**, 3-471
dextroamphetamine, 1-491, 2-4, 2-282, 2-286, 2-349
dextromethorphan (DXM, DM), 2-355
dextromoramide, 1-377, 2-75, 2-76, 3-492
  Palfium, 2-75, 3-492
dextropropoxyphene, 3-770
Dhanvantari, 2-24
diabetes, 1-121, 1-127, 1-137, 2-208, 2-339, 2-510, 3-52, 3-293, 3-335, 3-785
diabetes mellitus, 1-135, 1-291, 2-399
diacetylmorphine, see heroin
diacylglycerol, 1-257
Diagnostic and Statistical Manual of Mental Disorders (DSM), 1-25–1-27, 1-493, 2-26, 2-156–2-158, 2-219, 2-225, 2-381, 2-558, 2-559, 3-180, 3-228,

3-229, 3-240, 3-245, 3-247, 3-322–3-324, 3-326–3-328, 3-330–3-333, 3-335, 3-337, 3-402, 3-467, 3-522, 3-747, 3-750

Dial, *see* allobarbital

diallylbarbituric acid, *see* allobarbital

diaphragm, 1-41

diarrhea, 1-62, 1-147, 1-460, 2-16, 2-27, 2-38, 2-159, 2-329, 2-384, 2-415, 2-511, 2-525, 3-416

diazepam, 1-ix, 1-305, 1-323, 1-334, 1-352, 1-397, 1-421, 1-506, 1-507, 1-510, 2-13, 2-232–2-235, 2-237, 2-239, 2-311, 2-313, 2-559, 2-562, 3-213, 3-217, 3-238, 3-663

Valium, 1-506, 2-232, 2-233, 2-240, 2-311, 2-313, 3-137

diazepam binding inhibitor (DBI), 1-510

diazoxide, 3-661

dibenzepine, *see* dibenzipin

dibenzipin

dibenzepine, 2-135

dibenzoxazepine, 1-339

dibenzoxepine, 2-132

dibromogallic acid, 1-148

diclofenac, 3-299

Safeguard, 1-380, 3-145, 3-158, 3-161, 3-387

Diego, Dominican, 2-534

diencephalic nuclei, 2-67

diencephalon, 1-467

diethazine, 2-58

Diparcol, 2-58, 2-60–2-62

diethylbarbituric acid, *see* barbital

diethylene glycol (DEG), 3-48, 3-286

diethylketone, 1-142, 1-149

propionate, 1-142, 1-146, 1-149

diethylmalonilurate, *see* malonal

diethylmalonyl urea, *see* barbital

diethynyl ethylcarbonochloral, *see* dormiol

differential gel electrophoresis, 3-528, 3-559

diffusion, 1-17, 1-28, 1-111, 1-136, 1-262, 1-445, 2-486, 2-515, 3-137, 3-322, 3-620, 3-711, 3-712

digestion, 1-49, 1-120, 1-142, 2-494, 2-516, 2-532, 3-5, 3-559

digitaline, 1-119, 1-130, 2-276

Digitalis, 1-103, 1-104, 1-111, 1-119, 1-130, 1-138, 1-156, 1-160, 2-306, 2-328, 2-329, 2-545

Digitalis purpurea, 2-328

dihydrexidine, 3-652

DAR-0100, 3-652

dihydroergocornine, 2-545

dihydroergocriptine, 2-545

dihydroergocristine, 2-545

dihydroergotamine, 2-546

dihydromorphinone, 1-160

dihydropyrimidinase, 3-562, 3-563

Dilthey, Alfred, 2-269

dimerization, 1-263, 3-638

dimetacrine, 2-135

dimethoxymethane

methylal, 1-133, 1-139, 1-140, 1-144, 1-146, 1-151

dimethyltryptamine (DMT), 2-6, 2-486, 3-797

N,N-dimethyltryptamine, 3-797

dinitrile succinate, 2-4

dionine, *see* ethylmorphine

Dioscorides, 1-61, 2-413, 2-432, 2-458, 2-461, 2-472, 2-482, 2-492, 2-497, 2-506, 2-517

Diparcol, *see* diethazine

diphenhydramine (DPH, DHM), 2-144, 2-146, 3-67, 3-362, 3-466, 3-467, 3-762

Benadryl, 3-362, 3-762

diphenylhydantoin, *see* phenytoin

diphenylhydantoin sodium, *see* phenytoin
dipropylbarbituric acid, *see* propylbarbital
disease susceptibility, 1-288, 3-525
disulfiram, 2-17, 2-310, 2-311, 2-313, 2-
558, 3-329
Abstem, 2-311
Abstinyl, 2-311
Antabuse, 2-310, 2-311
Antiethyl, 2-311
Aversan, 2-311
Contralin, 2-311
Esperal, 2-311
Refusal, 2-311, 3-80, 3-81, 3-165
Stopetyl, 2-311
Temposil, 2-311
diuretic, 1-123, 1-144, 1-158, 1-346, 2-
490
divalproex sodium, *see* valproate
divalproic acid, *see* valproic acid
dizocilpine, 3-22, 3-23, **3-24**, 3-24–3-27,
3-642, 3-667
dizziness, 1-127, 1-158, 2-113, 2-159,
2-170, 2-171, 2-174, 2-247,
2-298, 2-299, 2-557
DMC, *see* norclozapine
DMI, *see* desipramine
DNA, *see* deoxyribonucleic acid (DNA)
DNA array, 1-282, 1-283, 3-547, *see also*
microarray
DNA methylation, 3-565
DNA microarray, 3-526, *see also*
microarray
DNA replication, 3-544
Dolatin, *see* meperidine
Dole, Vincent P., 2-308, 2-514
Dolophine, *see* methadone
Dolosal, *see* meperidine
Dolsa, Tomás, 3-720
Domenjoz, Robert, 2-126, 2-136, 3-9
Domeny, H., 1-127
Don Juan, 3-730

donepezil, 2-383–2-385, 2-388, 3-234
dopamine, 1-168, 1-237, 1-238, 1-240,
1-241, 1-243, 1-249, 1-255,
1-262, 1-268, 1-292, 1-311,
1-321, 1-340, 1-343, 1-358,
1-367–1-369, 1-399, 1-405,
1-459, 1-460, 1-466–1-472,
1-489, 1-491, 1-528–1-531,
2-17, 2-45, 2-46, 2-85, 2-88, 2-
93–2-99, 2-112, 2-142, 2-310,
2-311, 2-315, 2-351, 2-357,
2-402, 3-280, 3-402, 3-403,
3-459, 3-504–3-507, 3-510,
3-511, 3-517, 3-521, 3-525,
3-594, 3-598, 3-606, 3-611,
3-612, 3-625, 3-646, 3-648,
3-649, 3-653, 3-654, 3-659,
3-660, 3-664, 3-773
receptor, 1-238, 1-242, 1-277,
1-286, 1-295, 1-319, 1-445,
1-459, 1-470, 1-472, 2-17,
2-45, 2-46, 2-85, 2-94, 2-402,
3-247, 3-418, 3-472, 3-504,
3-506, 3-525, 3-610, 3-652
D_1, 1-238, 1-255, 1-268, 1-286,
1-312, 1-358, 1-369, 1-491,
1-492, 2-96, 2-97, 2-99, 3-27,
3-652
D_2, 1-238, 1-245, 1-286, 1-294,
1-312, 1-314, 1-319, 1-358,
1-369, 1-405, 1-445, 1-449,
1-472, 1-484, 1-491, 1-492,
2-46, 2-93, 2-95–2-99, 3-27,
3-504–3-506, 3-521, 3-585,
3-611, 3-648, 3-649, 3-651,
3-652, 3-654, 3-659, 3-660,
3-662
D_4, 1-238
dopamine agonist, 2-17
dopamine antagonist, 1-471, 2-100
dormiol, 1-148, 1-151, 1-158
amylene chloral, 1-148, 1-151
chloral amylene, 1-142

diethynyl ethylcarbonochloral, 1-151
dose-response relationship, 3-314
dosulepin, 1-339, 2-167
    dothiepin, 2-132, 2-135
    Prothiaden, 2-132, 2-167
Dover, Thomas, 2-414, 2-439, 2-508
Down syndrome, 1-290, 3-563
down-regulation, 1-450, 2-404, 3-514, 3-517, 3-518
Downame, John, 1-51
Dox, Arthur, 2-271
doxepin, 1-339, 1-357, 2-132, 2-135, 2-137, 2-175, 3-132, 3-457, 3-464, 3-466, 3-467
    Aponal, 2-132
    Sinequan, 2-132
doxorubicin, 3-473
Doyle, Arthur Conan, 3-497
Dr. Lepine, 1-148
Dreser, Heinrich, 2-416, 2-510, 3-193
dronabinol, *see* tetrahydrocannabinol (THC)
droperidol, 1-305, 1-318, 1-321, 2-81, 2-82, 3-472
    dehydrobenzperidol, 2-82
dropsy, 1-121, 1-123, 1-127, 1-144, 2-532, 3-327
drowning, 2-497, 3-740
drowsiness, 1-156, 1-322, 1-421, 2-8, 2-9, 2-29, 2-33, 2-38, 2-58, 2-79, 2-159, 2-175, 2-225, 2-260, 2-295, 2-546, 2-557, 3-6, 3-7, 3-491
drug addiction, 1-111, 1-113, 1-178, 1-406, 1-407, 2-281, 2-419, 2-448, 2-471, 2-484, 2-487, 3-15, 3-122, 3-185, 3-186, 3-190, 3-205, 3-563, 3-565, 3-723
drug development, 1-359, 1-361, 1-363, 1-367, 1-369, 2-226, 3-142, 3-256, 3-277

drug interactions, 1-357, 1-378, 1-379, 1-424, 2-12, 2-110, 2-115, 2-169, 2-171, 2-196, 2-562
drug tolerance, 3-665
drug toxicity, 3-48
du Bois-Reymond, Emil, 1-186
DU-125530, *see* alnespirone
Duboisia mioporcides, 1-133
Duboisia myoporoides, *see* Corkwood (Duboisia mioporcides)
duboisine, *see* hyoscyamine
duloxetine, 1-343, 2-168, 2-169, 2-173, 2-174, 2-176
    Cymbalta, 2-173
dura mater, 1-136
Dust, *see* phencyclidine
Dutch, 1-183, 1-376, 1-377, 2-439, 2-473, 3-64
dynamizing vital solution by Vindevogel, 1-144
dynorphin, 1-243, 1-287, 1-528
dysentery, 2-27, 2-414, 2-415, 2-516
dyskinesia, 1-295, 1-309, 1-311, 1-421, 2-17, 3-127, 3-135, 3-287, 3-474, 3-475
dyskinesias, 1-318, 2-38, 3-135
dyspepsia, 1-137, 1-145, 1-319, 2-38, 2-348, 2-456, 2-527
dyspnea, 1-150
dysthymic disorder, 3-327
dystonia, 1-284, 2-17

E

East India Company, 2-473, 2-532, 3-190
Easterfield, T.H., 2-519
Eberl, Irmfried, 3-94, 3-100
Ebers Papyrus, 2-413, 2-432, 2-433, 2-472
Ebn Baga, 3-440
Ebn Hazem, 3-440
Ebn Teimia, 3-440
Ebn-e-Khaldoun, 3-440

Eccles, John Carew, 1-205
eclampsia, 1-127, 1-147, 2-286, 2-448
Ecstasy, *see* MDMA (methylene-dioxymethamphetamine)
ECT, *see* electroconvulsive therapy (ECT)
edema, 1-443, 2-64, 3-215, 3-386
Edison, Thomas Alva, 2-527, 2-528
EEG, *see* electroencephalogram (EEG)
effector, 1-217, 1-224, 1-253, 1-262, 1-263, 1-510, 3-512
Effexor, *see* venlafaxine
efficacy, 1-x, 1-xxiv, 1-80, 1-98, 1-236, 1-264, 1-278, 1-294, 1-380, 1-383, 1-415, 1-416, 1-419–1-424, 1-429, 1-430, 1-471, 1-483, 1-485, 2-5, 2-9, 2-10, 2-34, 2-58, 2-59, 2-65, 2-93–2-98, 2-106, 2-108, 2-112, 2-114, 2-115, 2-129, 2-130, 2-132, 2-133, 2-135, 2-138, 2-141, 2-152, 2-154, 2-156, 2-157, 2-160, 2-167, 2-169–2-171, 2-173–2-176, 2-185, 2-189, 2-191, 2-193, 2-194, 2-196–2-198, 2-203, 2-205, 2-206, 2-208–2-211, 2-223, 2-225, 2-230, 2-233, 2-240, 2-246–2-248, 2-293, 2-294, 2-297, 2-299, 2-309, 2-314, 2-315, 2-354, 2-364, 2-383, 2-384, 2-391, 2-409, 2-555, 2-562, 3-12, 3-15, 3-25, 3-48–3-50, 3-165, 3-166, 3-234, 3-246, 3-255, 3-258, 3-277, 3-278, 3-281, 3-282, 3-285, 3-306–3-310, 3-312, 3-314–3-316, 3-327, 3-332–3-334, 3-364, 3-372, 3-373, 3-384, 3-387–3-390, 3-403, 3-471–3-476, 3-506, 3-514, 3-626, 3-628, 3-640–3-642, 3-645, 3-647–3-650, 3-652–3-654, 3-657, 3-659, 3-662, 3-664–3-668
Egas Moniz, António, 1-xxiv, 1-21, 2-341, 3-729
eglumegad
    LY-354740, 3-658, 3-668
ego, 1-11, 1-13, 1-17, 2-109, 2-159
Ehrenberg, Christian Gottfried, 1-190
Ehrlich, Paul, 1-169, 1-236, 1-419, 3-280, 3-582
Einhorn, Alfred, 2-456
Eisleb, O., 2-76
ejaculation, 3-13, 3-131
EKG, *see* electrocardiogram (EKG)
el-Gozia, Ebn el-Quuem, 3-440
Elavil, *see* amitriptyline
electrocardiogram (EKG), 3-299
electroconvulsive therapy (ECT), 1-xxiv, 1-xxviii, 1-479, 1-490, 2-33, 2-34, 2-63, 2-64, 2-69, 2-125, 2-126, 2-153, 2-185, 2-338, 2-340, 2-407, 2-532, 3-84, 3-172, 3-236, 3-282, 3-283, 3-331, 3-343–3-355, 3-358, 3-514, 3-523, 3-630, 3-636, 3-640, 3-645
electroencephalogram (EEG), 2-295, 2-296, 3-349, 3-641
electron microscopy, 1-169, 1-170, 1-206, 1-207, 2-235, 3-582
electron transport, 3-561
electrophoresis, 2-235, 3-527, 3-546, 3-550, 3-556
electroshock therapy, 1-309, 2-23, 2-272
Elephant, *see* phencyclidine
eliprodil, 3-643
Elixir Sulfanilamide, 1-418, 3-48
Elliot, Thomas R., 1-169
eltoprazine, 2-370
EMA, *see* European Medicines Agency (EMA)
Embalming Fluid, *see* phencyclidine
embryology, 1-188, 1-195
Emde, Hermann, 2-523

EMEA, *see* European Medicines Evaluation Agency (EMEA)

emetic, 1-62, 1-121, 1-123, 1-132, 1-410,
2-88, 2-305, 2-306, 3-473

EMIT, *see* enzyme-multiplied immunoassay technique (EMIT)

encephalitis, 2-38, 3-570

encephalopathy, 2-5, 2-40

Endicott, Jean, 3-324

endocrine system, 3-606

endocytosis, 3-516, 3-568

endogenous, 1-12, 1-20, 1-171, 1-242,
1-243, 1-245, 1-257, 1-286,
1-462, 1-471, 1-480, 1-510,
1-528–1-531, 2-6, 2-13, 2-108,
2-109, 2-115, 2-144, 2-167,
2-235, 2-236, 2-399, 2-420,
2-422–2-424, 2-461, 2-510,
3-245, 3-331, 3-348, 3-365,
3-386, 3-460, 3-505, 3-571,
3-586, 3-599, 3-645, 3-646,
3-656, 3-667, 3-745, 3-747,
3-770, 3-773

endomorphine-1, 2-422

endomorphine-2, 2-422
inhibits, 2-422

endomorphines, 2-422

endoplasmic reticulum, 1-257, 1-262

endorphin, 1-528, 2-510, 3-386, 3-598,
3-601, 3-610

Engel, George L., 2-398

enkephalin, 1-243, 1-528, 1-531, 2-422,
2-424, 3-645

enkephalins, 2-236, 2-422–2-424, 3-386,
3-645, 3-773

enteric, 2-192

Entralgo, Laín, 1-206

Entralgo, Pedro Laín, 1-38, 3-715–3-717,
3-731, 3-801

enuresis, 3-448, 3-461–3-464

enzyme, 1-235, 1-252, 1-255, 1-257,
1-259, 1-262, 1-267, 1-283,
1-293, 1-335, 1-340, 1-381,
1-384, 1-420, 1-451, 1-480,
1-488, 2-12, 2-106, 2-112,
2-169, 2-170, 2-285, 2-353,
2-390, 2-424, 2-544, 3-63,
3-506, 3-509, 3-511, 3-513,
3-550, 3-560, 3-569, 3-570,
3-584–3-586, 3-635, 3-641

enzyme-multiplied immunoassay technique (EMIT), 1-361, 1-381, 1-
382, 1-409

eosinophilia, 3-66

ephedra, 2-479, 2-523, 3-430
Ephedra vulgaris, 2-348, 3-796
Ma Huang, 2-523, 3-430

Ephedra vulgaris, *see* ephedra

ephedrine, 2-276, 2-286, 2-348, 2-349,
2-479, 2-515, 2-523, 3-796

epidermal necrolysis
toxic, 2-196

epidermis, 1-124

Epifanio, Giuseppe, 2-272

epilepsy, 1-43, 1-108, 1-126–1-128,
1-131, 1-132, 1-134, 1-136,
1-140–1-142, 1-144, 1-145,
1-147–1-149, 1-151, 1-152,
1-154, 1-157, 1-158, 1-160,
1-174, 1-262, 1-328, 1-333, 1-
379, 1-514, 2-10, 2-27, 2-191,
2-194, 2-203, 2-204, 2-208,
2-259–2-261, 2-266, 2-270,
2-277, 2-278, 2-329, 2-335,
2-363, 2-448, 2-454, 2-511,
2-517, 2-519, 2-521–2-524,
3-14, 3-90, 3-99, 3-133, 3-188,
3-343, 3-344, 3-347, 3-429,
3-430, 3-432, 3-462, 3-604,
3-607, 3-736, 3-740

epinephrine, 1-162, 1-171, 1-205, 1-234,
1-235, 1-241, 1-368, 1-462, 1-
466, 1-467, 1-488, 2-32, 2-357,
2-523, 3-598, 3-610, 3-762, 3-
764

Epling, Carl, 2-466

EPSP, *see* excitatory postsynaptic potential (EPSP)

Equanil, *see* meprobamate

Erasistratus, 1-184, 3-706, 3-733

Erasmus, 1-58, 1-59

ergobasine, *see* ergometrine

ergoloid
    Hydergine, 2-546

ergometrine
    ergobasine, 2-545

ergot, 1-130, 1-462, 1-463, 2-354, 2-356, 2-461–2-463, 2-484, 2-485, 2-543–2-545, 3-199, 3-594
    ergotism, 2-461, 2-543
    ergotoxine, 1-235, 2-544
    wheat horn, 2-543

ergotamine, 2-461, 2-535, 2-544, 2-545

ergotherapy, *see* lysergic acid diethylamide (LSD)

ergotoxine, *see* ergot

Erikson, Erik H., 3-729

erythrocyte, 1-284

erythroxyline, 2-526

Erythroxylon, *see* coca

Erythroxylon coca, *see* coca

Erythroxylum coca, *see* coca

escitalopram, 1-357, 1-360, 2-141, 2-157, 2-174
    Exodus, 2-490

eslicarbazepine, 2-210

esophagus, 1-41

Esperal, *see* disulfiram

Esquirol, Jean-Etienne-Dominique, *1-7*

Esquirol, Jean-Etienne-Dominique, 1-5, 1-6, 1-8, 1-93, 1-95–1-97, 1-105, 1-106, 2-521, 3-187, 3-321, 3-327, 3-736, 3-741, 3-742, 3-790

essential amino acid, 1-482, 2-144, 3-65

estragole, 3-796

estrogen, 1-268, 3-647

ethanol, 1-365, 1-465, 1-512, 2-6, 3-491, 3-494, 3-496

ethyl alcohol, 1-155, 1-505, 2-229, 3-201, 3-491–3-495

ethchlorvynol, 3-140

ether, 1-106, 1-108, 1-111, 1-133, 1-134, 1-147, 1-148, 1-150, 1-151, 1-305, 1-307, 1-322, 1-416, 2-220, 2-253, 2-438, 2-441–2-443, 2-446, 2-448, 2-449, 2-496, 2-505, 3-384, 3-491, 3-765

ethics, 1-xiii, 1-xxvii, 1-38, 3-38, 3-39, 3-79–3-82, 3-87–3-89, 3-101, 3-103, 3-104, 3-106–3-109, 3-122–3-127, 3-129, 3-137, 3-139, 3-141, 3-145, 3-153–3-155, 3-161–3-163, 3-165, 3-170, 3-225, 3-227, 3-238, 3-239, 3-249, 3-253, 3-256–3-258, 3-402, 3-728, 3-794

ethosuximide, 1-334, 2-209

ethoxycaffeine, 1-147

ethyl alcohol, *see* ethanol

ethyl chloride, 2-446, 2-448

ethyl-chloric-urethane, 1-149

ethylamphetamine, 3-55

ethylchloralurethane, 1-134

ethylmorphine, 2-307
    dionine, 1-146

eticyclidine, 3-22
    CI-400, 3-22
    PCE, 3-22

etiology, 1-11, 1-23, 1-26, 1-52, 1-162, 1-176, 1-178, 1-262, 1-393, 1-400, 2-96, 2-181, 2-348, 3-322, 3-326, 3-330–3-332, 3-335, 3-459, 3-467, 3-510, 3-522, 3-525, 3-661, 3-666

etomidate, 2-279, 3-350

etoperidone
    Staff, 1-309, 1-380, 2-79, 2-126, 2-129, 2-340, 3-9–3-11, 3-15, 3-53, 3-80, 3-232, 3-238, 3-364

etryptamine, *see α*-ethyltryptamine

eucalyptus phosphorus, 1-144

euforin, 1-151

eugenol, 3-796

European Medicines Agency (EMA), 3-51–3-53, 3-660

European Medicines Evaluation Agency (EMEA), 3-51, 3-65, 3-69, 3-660

evolution, 1-xxiii, 1-xxvi, 1-4, 1-11–1-13, 1-27, 1-49, 1-51, 1-53, 1-66, 1-91, 1-110, 1-154, 1-170, 1-172, 1-194, 1-207, 1-303, 1-305, 1-314, 1-527, 1-528, 1-530, 2-57, 2-61, 2-357, 2-449, 2-486, 2-487, 2-489, 2-505, 3-112, 3-141, 3-193, 3-208, 3-258, 3-284, 3-327, 3-329, 3-331, 3-335, 3-355, 3-371, 3-411, 3-416, 3-419, 3-456, 3-544, 3-559, 3-607, 3-723, 3-748, 3-766, 3-775

evolutionary theory, 1-9, 3-411–3-415, 3-419, 3-420

exalgine, 1-136, 1-147, 1-151

excitant, 1-119, 1-130, 1-133, 1-134, 1-143, 1-146, 1-154, 3-206, 3-596

excitatory amino acid, 3-460

excitatory neurotransmitter, 3-507, 3-598, 3-656

excitatory postsynaptic potential (EPSP), 3-600

existential, 1-20, 1-28, 3-283, 3-311, 3-712, 3-715, 3-745

exocytosis, 1-260

Exodus, *see* escitalopram

extension, 2-79, 2-160, 2-240, 2-298, 3-54, 3-97, 3-412, 3-419, 3-706, 3-712, 3-715, 3-742, 3-756

Ey, Henri, *1-20*, 1-21, 3-745, 3-750, 3-766, 3-790

eye diseases, 2-415, 2-506

ezogabine

retigabine, 2-210

F

Fabaceae, 3-797

face, 1-52, 1-96, 1-126, 1-132, 1-179, 1-397, 1-428, 2-39, 2-133, 2-154, 2-506, 3-84, 3-112, 3-254, 3-321, 3-405, 3-543, 3-587, 3-621

facet, 2-359, 3-153

facial paralysis, 3-63

fainting, 1-145

Falret, Jean-Pierre, 1-6, 1-14

fananserin, 2-97, 3-653

    RP-62204, 3-653

Faraday, Michael, 2-441

farampator

    ORG-24448, 3-658

Father Jofré, 3-707

Father Rousseau, 2-508

FDA, *see* Food and Drug Administration (FDA)

FDCA, *see* Federal Food, Drug, and Cosmetic Act (1938)

feces, 3-385

Federal Food, Drug, and Cosmetic Act (1938), 3-48

Feighner, John P., 1-26, 3-131, 3-132, 3-322, 3-324

felbamate, 1-329, 2-204, 3-299

Felipe, J., 2-458

femoxetine, 2-148

fenbutrazate, 3-67

fenclonine

    p-chloro-phenylalanine, 3-771

fenfluramine, 1-484, 1-493, 2-350, 2-524, **3-67**, 3-471

fenosol, 1-146

fenproporex, 3-67, 3-68

fentanyl, 1-305, 3-770

fermentation, 1-187, 2-489, 2-490, 2-492, 3-201, 3-434

Fernandez, Francisco Alonso, 3-723

Ferri, Enrico, 3-187
Ferrosol, 1-148
fertilization, 3-278
fetal alcohol syndrome, 3-188
fibromyalgia, 2-176, 2-210, 3-456, 3-474
Fink, Max, 3-351
First Psychiatrist, 1-8, 3-437
Fischer, Emil, 1-506, 2-105, 2-268, 2-531
Fischer, Eugen, 3-89
Fisher, Edmundo, 3-787, 3-789, 3-793
Fitzgerald, Francis Scott, 3-495
flesinoxan, 2-247, 2-370
Fleury, Tony Robert, 1-3, 1-84
fluanisone, 2-81
flumazenil, 1-369, 1-509, 1-511, 1-513,
        2-558, 3-499
    Ro 15-1788, 1-509
flunitrazepam, 1-363, 2-235, 2-293, 2-
        295, 2-297, 3-55, 3-213–3-217
    Rohypnol, 3-214
    roofies|hyperpage, 3-214
fluorescence polarization immunoas-
        say (FPIA), 1-361, 1-381,
        1-382
Fluothane, *see* halothane
fluotracene, 2-135
fluoxetine, 1-341, 1-343, 1-352, 1-
        356, 1-360, 1-423, 1-451,
        2-110, 2-141, 2-146–2-148,
        2-150–2-161, 2-168, 2-172,
        2-174–2-176, 2-197, 2-310,
        2-313, 3-132, 3-246, 3-251,
        3-313, 3-314, 3-453–3-456,
        3-464, 3-468, 3-471, 3-517,
        3-518, 3-562, 3-634, 3-640,
        3-642, 3-644, 3-646, 3-647,
        3-668
    Lilly 110140, 2-141, 2-148
    Prozac, 1-341, 1-423, 2-137, 2-141,
        2-310, 3-246
flupenthixol, 2-85, 2-88, 3-308, 3-309
fluphenazine, 1-311, 3-452
fluprazine, 2-370

flurazepam, 1-363, 1-397, 1-507, 2-293,
        2-295, 2-297, 3-217
    Dalmane, 1-507
fluroxene, 2-446
fluvoxamine, 1-341, 1-343, 1-352, 1-356,
        2-110, 2-141, 2-160, 2-172,
        2-175, 2-367, 3-132, 3-455,
        3-456, 3-464, 3-468, 3-645
Foerster, Otfrid, 1-206
folic acid deficiency, 1-334
Fonssagrives, J.B., 1-123
Fontana, Felice, 1-186
Fontanet, Pedro Mata, 3-741
Food and Drug Administration (FDA),
        1-323, 1-380, 1-385, 1-417, 1-
        420–1-424, 2-70, 2-81, 2-130,
        2-132, 2-133, 2-135, 2-137,
        2-141, 2-169, 2-187, 2-189,
        2-192, 2-193, 2-195–2-197,
        2-299, 2-309, 2-310, 2-312,
        2-481, 2-521, 3-14, 3-25, 3-48,
        3-51, 3-53, 3-81, 3-83, 3-113,
        3-180, 3-215, 3-239, 3-243,
        3-246, 3-248, 3-250, 3-252,
        3-310, 3-314, 3-388, 3-389,
        3-472, 3-649, 3-653, 3-793,
        3-794
    Psychopharmacologic Drugs Advi-
        sory Committee, 3-53
Food, Drug, and Insecticide Adminis-
        tration, 3-50
foot, 1-101
forebrain, 1-485
Foreest, Pieter van, 2-360
forensic psychiatry, 1-385, 3-748
Forestus, Petrus, 2-360
formaldehyde, 3-566, 3-598
    formalin, 2-76, 2-445
formalin, *see* formaldehyde
formanilide, 1-146
formic acid, 1-143, 2-88, 2-254, 2-257, 2-
        266
fosphenytoin, 1-332

fossa, 1-442, 3-187

Foucault, Michel, 1-3, 1-7, 1-23

Fourneau, Ernest, 1-152, 1-307, 2-56, 3-594

Fox, Herbert, 2-12, 2-105

FPIA, *see* fluorescence polarization immunoassay (FPIA)

fractures, 1-121, 2-338, 3-131
    bone, 3-349

Frank, Jerome David, 3-305

Frankel, S., 1-155

Frederick the Great, 2-532

Frenquel, *see* azacyclonol

Freud
    concaine, 2-477, 3-3

Freud, Anna, 1-21

Freud, Sigmund, 1-xxiv, 1-11, 1-14–1-17, *1-17*, 1-18, 2-305, 2-348, 2-404, 2-445, 2-456, 2-477, 2-529, 3-3, 3-316, 3-322, 3-327, 3-332, 3-383, 3-398, 3-497, 3-503, 3-711, 3-712, 3-742, 3-747, 3-748

Freyhan, Fritz A., 2-9

Friedreich, Johann Baptiste, 1-101

Friedrich, 1-101, 1-191, 2-439, 2-509, 2-510, 3-97, 3-741

Friedrich, Eduard, 3-593

Frobenius, W.G., 2-441

frontal, 1-xxiv, 1-220, 1-293, 1-444, 1-448, 1-451, 1-491, 2-341, 2-343, 2-372, 3-174, 3-349, 3-399, 3-401, 3-402, 3-517, 3-520, 3-527, 3-563, 3-634, 3-636, 3-645, 3-646, 3-653, 3-662, 3-773

Fuentenebro, Filiberto, 3-749

Fulton, John Farquhar, 2-342

Furshpaan, E.J., 1-170

G

G protein, 1-243, 1-245, 1-250, 1-252, 1-254, 1-255, 1-257, 1-268, 1-269, 1-280, 1-281, 1-285, 1-286, 1-292, 3-461, 3-509, 3-512, 3-514, 3-516–3-518, 3-520, 3-521, 3-523, 3-524, 3-527, 3-583, 3-598, 3-600, 3-605, 3-606, 3-610, 3-630, 3-633

G protein-activated inwardly rectifying K^+ channels (GIRK), 3-514

G protein-coupled receptor (GPCR), 1-263, 1-286, 1-287, 1-506, 3-516–3-518, 3-583, 3-584, 3-633

G protein-coupled receptor kinase (GRK), 3-517, 3-526

$G\alpha$, 1-255, 1-257

G. Washington, 2-484

G.J. Sarwar-Forner, 2-41

G22355, *see* imipramine

GABA, *see* γ-aminobutyric acid (GABA)

GABA$_A$ receptor
    GABA-benzodiazepine ionophore channel of chloride, 3-662
    GABA-benzodiazepine receptor, 2-298, 3-207, 3-625, 3-663, 3-664

GABA-benzodiazepine ionophore channel of chloride, *see* GABA$_A$ receptor

GABA-benzodiazepine receptor, *see* GABA$_A$ receptor

gabapentin, 1-329, 1-379, 2-206, 2-207, 2-209, 2-210, 3-452, 3-664

Gabor, Dennis, 1-228

Gaddum, J.H., 1-171

Gaedcke, Friedrich, 2-526

galantamine, 2-383, 2-384, 2-387

Galen, 1-39, 1-42, 1-43, 1-45–1-50, 1-74, 1-168, 1-184, 1-186, 1-335, 2-334, 2-413, 2-414, 2-432, 2-460, 2-461, 2-472, 2-482, 2-506, 2-511, 2-517, 3-94, 3-377, 3-706, 3-732

Galileo, 1-64

Gall, Franz Josef, 3-187
gallobromol, 1-138, 1-148
Galvani, Luigi, 1-168, 1-186, 3-593
gambling, 1-530
Gamgee, Arthur, 2-255
gamma vinyl-GABA (GVG), *see* vigaba-trin
Ganadol kandol, 1-147
Gandhi, Mahatma, 1-460
ganglion, 1-194, 1-196, 1-199, 1-264
ganglioplegic, 2-66, 2-67
gantenerumab, GSK933776A and BAN2401, 2-391
García-Valdecasas, Francisco, 2-32, 3-757, 3-760
Gardner, Russell, 3-417
garlic, 1-51, 3-430
Garma, Ángel, 3-711, 3-712, 3-731
Garofalo, Raffaele, 3-187
Garrabé, Jean, 1-28
Garrod, Alfred Baring, 2-184, 2-260
gas chromatography (GC), 1-359, 1-361, 1-362, 1-377, 1-381
gas chromatography-mass spectrom-etry (GC-MS), 1-359, 1-362, 1-365, 1-381, 1-382
gastritis, 2-527
gastrointestinal tract, 1-319, 2-222, 3-471
gates, 1-304
Gaubil, Antoine, 1-66
Gautier, Théophile, 2-484, 2-518, 3-492, 3-497
GC, *see* gas chromatography (GC)
Gedeon Richter, 3-651
Gelineau syrup, 1-144
Gelsemium, 1-129, 1-134, 1-146
    Gelsemium tincture , 1-151
Gelsemium sempervirens, 1-148
Gelsemium tincture , *see* Gelsemium
gene expression, 1-224, 1-226, 1-253, 1-260, 1-265, 1-282, 1-283, 1-292, 1-295, 1-451, 1-531,

3-513, 3-520, 3-526, 3-527, 3-546–3-548, 3-550–3-553, 3-565, 3-566, 3-568, 3-569, 3-610, 3-630, 3-631, 3-634, 3-635, 3-640, 3-661
general anesthetic, 2-4, 2-278, 3-23, 3-215, 3-216, 3-350
general anxiety disorder (GAD), 1-280, 2-246, 2-247, 3-664, 3-666
general hospital, 1-4, 1-8, 1-60, 1-62, 2-29, 2-443, 3-207, 3-218, 3-352, 3-707, 3-715, 3-718, 3-722
general paresis, 1-105, 1-108, *see also* dementia
genetic diseases, 1-399, 3-603
genetic heterogeneity, 1-291
genomics, 1-179, 1-278, 1-282, 1-283, 1-289, 1-295, 3-526–3-528, 3-544, 3-546, 3-553, 3-554, 3-567
gentiana
    gentian extract, 1-138
    gentian root, 1-138
Gerais, Minas, 3-798
Gerard, John, 2-438
Giné y Partagás, Juan, 3-719, 3-741, 3-742
Ginestet, D., 2-34
gingival hyperplasia, 1-332
Ginkgo biloba, 1-359
gland, 1-143, 1-168, 2-397, 3-5
glaucoma, 2-520
GlaxoWellcome, 1-319
Globe of Flowers Cough Syrup, 2-528
glucocorticoid, 1-268, 1-399, 2-397, 2-401, 2-408, 3-633, 3-640, 3-646
glucose, 1-161, 1-260, 1-267, 1-451, 1-481, 1-493, 2-59, 2-63, 2-248, 2-306, 2-340, 2-401, 3-349, 3-402, 3-561, 3-769
glutamatergic, 1-292, 1-404, 1-405, 1-530, 1-531, 2-93, 2-98, 2-99,

2-387, 2-388, 3-507–3-509, 3-563, 3-609, 3-643, 3-644, 3-655, 3-656, 3-658, 3-659, 3-667

glutethimide, 1-331, 2-363, 3-763

glycerol, 2-11

glycogen, 1-267, 3-512

glycosylation, 1-252, 3-553

gnoscopine, 2-416

Goddard, Henry, 3-188

Goerden, 3-99

Goffman, Erving, 1-23

Goglia, Gabriel, 1-159

goiter, 2-448

Goldstein, 1-85–1-87, 1-95, 1-243, 2-420, 3-747

Golgi, 1-169, 1-190–1-196, 1-201, 2-14

Goring, Charles, 3-188

gout, 1-416, 2-7, 2-184, 2-439, 2-506, 2-532, 3-14, 3-439

Gowers, William Richard, 2-259

Goyanes, Juan José Barcia, 3-715, 3-717

GPCR, see G protein-coupled receptor (GPCR)

Gracia, Diego, 3-731

Graf, Herbert, 1-16

Graf, Otto, 2-258

Grageas G, 1-144

Grageas Gelineau, 1-144

Grasset, Joseph, 1-14

Graves' disease, 1-133

gray matter, 1-139, 1-143, 1-149, 1-199, 1-444, 1-445, 1-451

Greatrakes, Valentine, 3-380

Gregoretti, L., 2-537

Grien, Hans Baldung, 2-435

Griesinger, Wilhelm, 1-11, 1-12, 1-105, 2-266, 2-496, 2-501, 2-513, 3-187, 3-322, 3-736

Griffith, Harold Randall, 2-447

Grigor, John, 2-518

group size, 1-431

growth hormone, 1-489, 1-492, 2-399, 3-215, 3-331

Guachamaca, 1-133

guaiacum, 1-62

Guiraud, Paul, 2-58, 2-59

Gupta, J.C., 2-30

gut, 2-14

Gutiérrez, Emilio Cabello, 1-132

Guttfreund, Daniel G., 3-730

gymnemic acid, 1-142

gyrus, 1-485, 2-153, 3-401

H

Häfliger, F., 2-126

Haase, H.J., 2-39

Hadamar, 1-xxv, 3-97

Hadamarius, 1-xxv

haematoxylin
    hematoxylin, 1-190

Hague Convention of 1912, see opium

hair, 1-361, 1-362, 1-377, 2-160, 2-438, 3-376, 3-740

Hakim, 2-10, 2-32, 3-439

Hakim, R.A., 2-32

Halcion, see triazolam

Hald, Jens, 2-311

Haller, Albrecht von, 1-186, 2-3

hallucinations, 1-6, 1-18, 1-118, 1-120, 1-140, 1-142, 1-155, 1-326, 1-341, 2-26, 2-219, 2-267, 2-273, 2-337, 2-340, 2-355, 2-357, 2-434, 2-448, 2-484, 2-513, 2-530, 3-64, 3-135, 3-206, 3-215, 3-346, 3-432, 3-499, 3-505, 3-507, 3-594, 3-611, 3-742, 3-749, 3-797

hallucinogen, 1-162, 1-401, 1-406, 1-462, 1-471, 2-15, 2-316, 2-348, 2-354, 2-355, 2-434, 2-446, 2-447, 2-449, 2-462, 2-471, 2-484–2-486, 2-533, 2-536, 2-538, 3-54, 3-205, 3-210, 3-498, 3-606

hallucinogens, 2-356
haloperidol, 1-316, 1-358, 1-361, 1-381,
    1-383, 1-449, 1-451, 1-468,
    1-470, 1-471, 2-13, 2-17, 2-41,
    2-75–2-77, 2-79–2-82, 2-88,
    2-94, 2-210, 2-365, 3-134,
    3-278, 3-308–3-310, 3-472,
    3-649, 3-652, 3-653, 3-659,
    3-661, 3-773
    R 1625, 2-79, 2-80
halothane, 1-306, 2-446
    Fluothane, 2-446
Halsted, William, 2-478
Halsted, William S., 2-445, 2-529
Hamill, Owen, 1-172
hand, 1-12–1-14, 1-19, 1-24, 1-27, 1-28,
    1-41, 1-46, 1-49, 1-51, 1-57,
    1-74, 1-90, 1-97, 1-108, 1-128,
    1-155, 1-156, 1-198, 1-228,
    1-233, 1-236, 1-314, 1-447,
    1-449, 1-466, 1-484, 1-491–
    1-493, 2-7, 2-42, 2-58, 2-80,
    2-147, 2-159, 2-205, 2-220,
    2-225, 2-246, 2-249, 2-283,
    2-296, 2-313, 2-383, 2-404,
    2-432, 2-436, 2-438, 2-439,
    2-441, 2-442, 2-448, 2-458,
    2-471, 2-476, 2-481, 2-513,
    2-517, 2-525, 3-42, 3-57, 3-82,
    3-84, 3-122, 3-128–3-130,
    3-170, 3-176, 3-189, 3-205,
    3-207, 3-211, 3-218, 3-226,
    3-227, 3-251, 3-291, 3-296,
    3-310, 3-323, 3-328, 3-333,
    3-350, 3-368, 3-402, 3-419,
    3-454, 3-466, 3-526, 3-545,
    3-570, 3-571, 3-582, 3-594,
    3-598, 3-603, 3-621, 3-636,
    3-642, 3-644, 3-646, 3-647,
    3-667, 3-717, 3-728, 3-738,
    3-750, 3-765
Hare, Hobart, 2-519
Harl, Jean Marie, 2-65

harmal
    wild rue, 3-430
harmine, 1-462, 2-445
Harris, Titus H., 2-40
Harrison Narcotics Tax Act (1914), 3-192
Harvey, William, 1-64, 2-532, see also
    coffee
Hasan-Ibn-al-Sabbah, 2-483
hashish, see cannabis
Hauptmann, Alfred, 1-328, 2-261, 2-276
hay fever, 2-58, 2-527
Hayyan, Jabber Ebn, 3-437
head, 1-12, 1-18, 1-48, 1-82, 1-88, 1-93,
    1-120, 1-121, 1-123, 1-134,
    1-186, 2-131, 2-133, 2-156,
    2-167, 2-174, 2-184, 2-326,
    2-331–2-333, 2-335, 3-9, 3-94,
    3-193, 3-364, 3-381, 3-715,
    3-743, 3-760, 3-772, 3-787,
    3-792
headache, 2-176, 2-259, 2-298, 2-299, 3-
    379, 3-430, 3-432, 3-474
health administration, 3-122, 3-139, 3-
    299
Healy, David, 2-39, 2-70, 3-144, 3-359
heart, 1-xvi, 1-xvii, 1-41, 1-44, 1-48,
    1-50, 1-52, 1-97, 1-126, 1-127,
    1-132, 1-136, 1-138, 1-141,
    1-145, 1-152, 1-153, 1-155–
    1-157, 1-167, 1-184, 1-205,
    1-234, 1-235, 1-421, 1-424,
    1-449, 1-466, 2-29, 2-79, 2-80,
    2-150, 2-225, 2-285, 2-511,
    3-514, 3-641, 3-738, 3-743
heart failure, 2-329
Heffter, A., 2-534
Heidegger, Martin, 1-19, 3-712, 3-729
Heidelberg, 2-254, 3-92, 3-717
Heinroth, Johann Christian August,
    1-11, 1-101
Heinze, Gerardo, 3-801
Heinze, Hans, 3-99
Heister, Lorenz, 2-441

hellebore, 1-42, 1-49, 1-61, 1-62, 1-68, 1-90, 1-97, 2-325, 2-327, 3-492
  black hellebore, 1-42, 2-359
  Helleborus niger, 2-359
Helleborus niger, *see* hellebore
Helmont, Jan Baptist van, 1-65, 2-439
hematoporphyrin, 2-4
hematoxylin, *see* haematoxylin
hemorrhoids, 2-506
hemp, *see* cannabis
henbane, 1-119, 1-140, 1-147, 1-151, 2-3, 2-265, 2-361, 2-432–2-434, 2-436, 2-438, 2-439, 2-447–2-449, 2-506, 3-185, 3-499
  henbane juice, 2-436
  henbane oil, 1-151
  Hyoscyamus niger, 1-155, 2-361, 2-433, 2-447
henbane juice, *see* henbane
henbane oil, *see* henbane
Henle, Jacob, 1-187
hepatitis, 2-418
hepatitis C, 3-569, 3-646
Hera, 1-61, 2-325
Hernandez, Francisco, 2-534
heroin, 1-530, 2-308–2-310, 2-316, 2-328, 2-416, 2-419, 2-453, 2-475, 2-476, 2-478, 2-487, 2-505, 2-507, 2-510, 2-514, 2-560, 3-54, 3-83, 3-189, 3-190, 3-192, 3-195–3-197, 3-199, 3-205, 3-209
  Afghan, Thai, 2-487
  dependence, 2-315, 2-419, 2-513–2-515, 3-196, 3-211
  dependence treatment, 2-315
  diacetylmorphine, 2-507, 2-510, 3-193
  discovery, 2-510
  from morphine, 2-453
  Heroina, 3-195
  Horse, 1-159, 2-497
  prescription, 2-419
Heroina, *see* heroin
Herophilos of Chalcedon, 1-184
herpes simplex, 3-568
Hesiod, 2-472
Hesse, H., 2-534
heterocyclic antidepressants, 3-327
hexobarbital, 1-160, 1-465, 2-278, 2-279, 2-283
  Narcosan, 2-307
Heyde, Werner, 3-94
Hickman, Henry Hill, 2-442
high performance liquid chromatography (HPLC), 1-174, 1-359, 1-361, 1-362, 1-365, 1-367, 1-378, 1-381, 1-382
high-performance liquid chromatography-mass spectrometry (HPLC-MS), 1-359
high-throughput screening, 1-287, 1-351
high-throughput screening (HTS), 1-351, 3-585
Hill, Austin Bradford, 3-87
Hippocrates, 1-xvii, 1-38, 1-45, 1-68, 1-167, 2-405, 2-413, 2-458, 2-461, 2-463, 2-472, 2-484, 2-506, 2-511, 3-77, 3-124, 3-332, 3-377, 3-732
Hippocratic, 1-38, 1-43, 1-61, 1-73, 2-359, 3-77, 3-101, 3-106, 3-125, 3-155, 3-241, 3-705, 3-706
Hippocratic Oath, 3-87, 3-103, 3-124–3-126, 3-155
Hippocratism, 1-xxvi, 1-73
Hirsch, August, 1-100
His, Wilhelm, 1-193
histamine, 1-286, 1-357, 2-56, 2-158, 2-406, 3-6, 3-361, 3-464, 3-561, 3-600, 3-655
histology, 1-183, 1-188, 1-191, 1-196, 3-742

Hitler, Adolf, 3-90, 3-91, 3-93, 3-94

Hobson, James Allan, 1-xxvii

Hoffer, Abram, 2-311, 2-536, 3-792

Hoffman, 2-545

Hoffmann, H., 1-11

Hoffmann, Hermann, 3-92

Hofmann, 2-432, 2-535, 2-538, 2-545–2-547, 2-552

Hofmann, Albert, 2-96, 2-447, 2-462, 2-464, 2-466, 2-485, 2-535, 2-544, 2-545, 2-547, 2-551, 3-199, 3-594

Hog, *see* phencyclidine

Holmes, Oliver Wendell, 2-431

Holmes, Sherlock, 3-497

Holy Land, 2-461, 2-472

Holzinger, O., 2-126

homeostasis, 1-214, 1-215, 1-226, 1-488, 2-61, 2-397, 3-336

Homer, 2-434, 2-451, 2-490, 2-516, 3-492, 3-499

homovanillic acid, 1-491, 3-504, 3-649

Honore, Saint, 1-143

Hooke, Robert, 1-183, 1-186, 2-449

Hooker, Worthington, 3-126

Hoppe-Seyler, Felix, 2-254

Horace, 2-272, 3-494, 3-499

hordenine, 2-535, *see also* peyote
Peyocactin, 2-535

hormone, 1-268, 1-285, 1-331, 1-463, 1-481, 2-397, 3-4, 3-635, 3-640, 3-642, 3-769

Horn, Ernst, 1-103

Horse, *see* heroin

Horton, Richard, 3-249

Hotopf, Matthew, 2-138

HPLC, *see* high performance liquid chromatography (HPLC)

Hua To, 3-432

Huette, Charles, 2-258

Hughes, John, 1-242, 2-422

Huguenard, Pierre, 2-61

Hui, Wai Mo, 3-465

Humboldt, Alexander von, 2-526

Husen, Hermann von, 2-270

Husquet, H., 1-158

Hussar, H.E., 2-38

Huxley, Aldous, 1-322, 2-222, 2-464, 2-486, 3-498, 3-499

Huxley, Andrew F., 1-172

hydantoin, 1-160, 1-328

Hydergine, *see* ergoloid

Hydrastis canadensis, 1-130

hydrazine, 1-340, 2-7, 2-12, 2-105, 2-108, 2-110, 2-114

hydrochlorate, 1-119

hydrochloric ether, 1-129, 1-146

hydrochlorothiazide (HCT, HCTZ, HZT), 3-299

hydrocortisone
cortisol, 1-268, 1-399, 1-484, 1-490, 1-496, 3-331, 3-522, 3-640, 3-642, 3-646, 3-667, 3-775

hydrolysis, 1-255, 1-259, 2-87, 2-88, 2-382

hydrophobic, 3-558, 3-559, 3-586

hydroquinone, 1-147

hydrotherapy, 1-xxiv, 1-15, 1-118, 1-137, 1-140, 2-331, 2-332, 2-364

hydroxydione, 2-279

hydroxylation, 1-339, 1-383, 2-106, 2-152

hydroxyzine, 1-326, 2-248, 2-249, 3-467

hyoscine, *see* scopolamine

hyoscyamine, 1-147, 1-155, 2-4, 2-266, 2-328, 2-434, 2-445, 2-448, 2-449
daturine, 1-119, 1-130
duboisine, 1-133, 1-136, 1-148

hyoscyamine bromhydrate, 1-160

Hyoscyamus niger, *see* henbane

hyperalgesia, 3-460, 3-473

hyperbilirubinemia
neonatal, 2-286

hyperesthesia, 1-131

hyperforin, 1-358, 1-364–1-367, 1-370, 3-583

hyperglycemia, 3-661

hyperhidrosis, 3-315

Hypericaceae, 1-364, 2-458

hypericin, 1-358, 1-364–1-366, 2-458

Hypericum perforatum, 1-364, 2-458, 3-584

hyperpolarization, 3-662

hyperprolactinemia, 2-98

hypersensitivity, 1-238, 1-397, 1-489, 1-492

hypertension, 1-341, 1-460, 2-10, 2-29, 2-35, 2-38, 2-40, 2-110, 2-174, 2-309, 3-307, 3-335, 3-661
  pulmonary, 3-67, 3-471

hyperthyroidism, 3-763

hypertonic, 2-59

hyperventilation, 2-275

hypnal, 1-139, 1-140, 1-147, 1-151

hypnoacetine, 1-150

hypnoacetylene, 1-146

Hypnone, see acetophenone

hypnopyrine, 1-150

hypnotic, 1-xxv, 1-xxvii, 1-110, 1-118, 1-119, 1-123, 1-127, 1-131–1-136, 1-138, 1-139, 1-141, 1-142, 1-144, 1-146–1-151, 1-154–1-160, 1-305, 1-308, 1-322–1-324, 1-328, 1-329, 1-331, 1-334, 1-336, 1-352, 1-361, 1-377, 1-410, 1-460, 1-506, 2-4, 2-28, 2-32, 2-40, 2-56, 2-58, 2-61, 2-63, 2-65, 2-66, 2-79, 2-81, 2-111, 2-126, 2-220, 2-233, 2-236, 2-239, 2-254, 2-256, 2-265–2-270, 2-272, 2-273, 2-276–2-279, 2-283, 2-285, 2-286, 2-293–2-295, 2-297–2-299, 2-349, 2-361, 2-363, 2-448, 2-455, 2-519, 2-524, 2-555, 2-557, 3-8, 3-10, 3-49, 3-64, 3-65, 3-67, 3-140, 3-180, 3-189, 3-210, 3-214, 3-216–3-218, 3-277, 3-364, 3-365, 3-384, 3-475, 3-491, 3-496, 3-594, 3-604, 3-605, 3-665, 3-685, 3-711, 3-798, 3-800

hypodermic treatment, 1-144

hypoglycemia, 2-364, 3-666

hypokinesia, 1-467

hyponatremia, 2-209

hypotension, 1-153, 1-345, 2-67, 2-150, 2-159, 2-285, 2-309, 2-521, 2-524
  orthostatic, 2-67, 2-113, 3-131, 3-474

hypothalamus, 1-220–1-223, 1-225, 1-226, 1-287, 1-408, 1-409, 1-466, 2-153, 2-397, 3-563, 3-598, 3-645

hypothyroidism, 2-402

hypoxia, 2-354, 3-604, 3-666

hysteria, 1-14–1-16, 1-44, 1-45, 1-73, 1-108, 1-121, 1-126–1-128, 1-131, 1-132, 1-136, 1-137, 1-140, 1-141, 1-144, 1-145, 1-149, 1-151, 2-59, 2-448, 2-519, 2-527, 2-532, 3-332, 3-343, 3-344, 3-432, 3-712

I

Ibn-Sina, 3-732

iboga, 2-445, see also ibogaine
  Tabernanthe iboga, 2-316

ibogaine, 2-316, 2-445

ibotenic acid, 2-449

ICH, see International Conference on Harmonisation (ICH)

ICT, see insulin coma therapy

Ideler, Karl Wilhelm, 1-11, 1-101

ifenprodil, 3-643

iloperidone, 2-98, 3-649

imidazenil, 3-663

iminodibenzyl, 2-7, 2-12, 2-126, 3-9, 3-10, 3-12
imipramine, 1-ix, 1-22, 1-178, 1-240, 1-241, 1-336, 1-337, 1-339, 1-357, 1-361, 1-383, 1-421, 1-422, 1-479, 2-7, 2-12, 2-13, 2-16, 2-109, 2-110, 2-113, 2-125, 2-129, 2-130, 2-132, 2-133, 2-135–2-137, 2-142, 2-146, 2-156–2-158, 2-160, 2-171, 2-172, 2-174, 2-191, 2-407, 3-3, **3-9**, 3-11, 3-12, 3-15, 3-130–3-132, 3-277, 3-278, 3-282, 3-332, 3-350, 3-365, 3-366, 3-368, 3-448, 3-452–3-454, 3-462, 3-463, 3-467, 3-504, 3-628, 3-634, 3-642, 3-645, 3-668, 3-765, 3-766, 3-769, 3-770
    discovery of, 1-421, 3-364, 3-367, 3-369
    G22355, 2-12, 2-13, 2-127, 3-10, 3-11, 3-365
    synthesis of, 1-352
    Tofranil, 1-479, 2-128, 3-11, 3-12, 3-366
immunization, 2-390, 2-391, 3-285
immunoassay, 1-359, 1-377, 1-381
immunological, 1-510, 2-402, 2-404, 3-63, 3-64, 3-645, 3-646, 3-787
Imovane, *see* zopiclone
implantation, 1-18
impotence, 1-144, 1-145, 1-328, 2-259, 2-517, 3-300
in vitro, 1-172, 1-242, 1-283, 1-285, 1-362, 1-363, 1-447, 1-450, 2-142, 2-144, 2-169, 2-235, 2-388, 3-513, 3-558, 3-568, 3-570, 3-571, 3-583, 3-585, 3-646, 3-773
in vivo, 1-174, 1-242, 1-259, 1-359, 1-367–1-369, 1-441, 1-447, 1-450, 1-483, 2-94, 2-96–2-98,
2-144, 2-150, 2-152, 2-169, 2-235, 2-266, 2-298, 2-425, 3-384, 3-505, 3-566, 3-568, 3-571, 3-583, 3-600, 3-609, 3-648, 3-659
incarceration, 1-xv, 1-4, 2-315, 2-514, 3-205, 3-211, 3-235, 3-744
indalpine, 2-148
Indian hemp, *see* cannabis
infantile convulsions, 1-140
infantile sexuality, 1-16
infectious disease, 1-153, 2-338
infertility, 3-738
inflammation
    arachnoiditis, 1-105
influenza, 1-143, 1-153, 2-404, 3-63
informed consent, 1-xxvii, 1-415, 1-419, 1-422, 3-80, 3-88, 3-90, 3-101, 3-104, 3-105, 3-108, 3-111, 3-112, 3-133, 3-135, 3-136, 3-153, 3-156–3-159, 3-164–3-166, 3-169–3-172, 3-174, 3-178, 3-181, 3-237, 3-252, 3-386
ingestion, 1-94, 1-127, 1-134, 1-135, 1-404, 1-510, 2-110, 2-240, 2-462, 2-485, 2-513, 2-543, 3-131, 3-277, 3-279, 3-603
inhibitory postsynaptic potential, 3-600
    IPSP, 3-600
inositol, 1-257, 1-259, 1-447, 2-248, 2-249, 3-606
insanity, 1-4–1-9, 1-11, 1-25, 1-59, 1-62, 1-79, 1-80, 1-82–1-87, 1-89, 1-95, 1-97–1-100, 1-104, 1-106–1-108, 1-112, 1-460, 2-10, 2-229, 2-325, 2-326, 2-328–2-332, 2-338, 2-363, 2-405, 2-496, 2-510, 2-513, 2-521, 2-522, 3-154, 3-187, 3-188, 3-280, 3-283, 3-438, 3-439, 3-708, 3-717, 3-744
insertion, 1-264, 1-295

insomnia, 1-93, 1-120, 1-121, 1-124, 1-127, 1-131–1-145, 1-148, 1-149, 1-151–1-153, 1-156–1-159, 1-324, 1-352, 1-421, 2-4, 2-27, 2-59, 2-159, 2-171, 2-174, 2-176, 2-233, 2-239, 2-260, 2-266, 2-270, 2-285, 2-293–2-299, 2-351, 2-438, 2-454, 2-455, 2-511, 2-513, 2-518, 2-524, 2-555, 2-557, 2-562, 3-64, 3-65, 3-67, 3-214, 3-215, 3-468, 3-475, 3-476, 3-496, 3-652, 3-662, 3-740, 3-796

inspiration, 1-462, 2-451, 2-490, 3-359

Institut Pasteur, 1-307, 2-56, 2-126, 3-6, 3-594

insula, 1-451

insulin, 1-ix, 1-19, 1-21, 2-306, 2-339, 2-340, 2-405, 3-4, 3-344, 3-347, 3-384, *see also* pepetide hormones

insulin coma, *see* insulin coma therapy

insulin coma therapy, 1-xxiv, 2-5, 2-125, 2-307, 2-326, 2-364

criticism of, 2-340

ICT, 2-5

insulin coma, 2-325, 2-340, 2-341, 3-282, 3-344

insulin shock, 2-276, 2-405, 2-407, 3-344

insulin receptor, 1-267, 3-570

insulin resistance, 2-401

insulin shock, *see* insulin coma therapy

insulin shock therapy, 2-272

International Conference of Psychopharmacology, 2-68

International Conference on Harmonisation (ICH), 3-54, 3-101, 3-106, 3-107

International Drug Control Program, 2-471

International Narcotics Control Board, 2-471, 3-54, 3-196, 3-209

International Opium Convention, *see* opium

International Statistical Classification of Diseases and Related Health Problems, 3-325

interneurons, 1-224, 1-225, 1-227, 2-11

internexin, 3-563

intestinal colics, 2-448

intracranial hypertension, 3-352

intraocular pressure, 2-447, 2-520

intravascular hemolysis, 3-64

intravenous anesthetic, 2-279

intussusception, 1-187

inversion, 3-202, 3-331

ion, 1-172, 1-205, 1-252, 1-254, 1-255, 1-257, 1-260, 1-262, 1-268, 1-284, 1-286, 1-307, 2-239, 2-260, 3-434, 3-507, 3-512, 3-556, 3-557, 3-559, 3-585, 3-587, 3-598, 3-600, 3-601, 3-604, 3-605, 3-609, 3-662

ionization, 3-556, 3-560

Ipomoea violacea, 2-465, 2-538

ipral, 1-160

iprindole, 2-132, 2-135, 3-644

Prondol, 2-132

iproniazid, 1-ix, 1-22, 1-177, 1-340, 1-352, 1-357, 1-384, 1-419, 1-420, 1-422, 1-466, 1-479, 1-480, 2-7, 2-12, 2-15, 2-44, 2-105–2-107, 2-110, 2-125, 2-407, 3-278, 3-282, 3-366, **3-367**, 3-367, 3-368, 3-504, 3-765, 3-774

Marsilid, 1-479

ipsapirone, 1-326, 1-484, 2-246

IPSP, *see* inhibitory postsynaptic potential

iris, 1-122

iron oxysaccharate, 1-148

iron valerianate, 1-147

irritable bowel syndrome, 3-461

ischemia, 2-286, 2-389, 3-22, 3-25, 3-666

Isidore of Seville, 1-43, 3-706, 3-732

isocarboxazid, 1-340, 1-341, 2-12, 2-107, 2-110, 3-765

isoenzymes, 2-111, 2-114, 2-168

isoflurane, 2-446

isoniazid, 1-340, 1-352, 1-377, 1-384, 2-12, 2-15, 2-105–2-107, 3-278, 3-367, 3-368

isotope-coded affinity tag (ICAT), 3-556, 3-559

ispronicline
    AZD3480, 3-655

Itallie, E.I. van, 2-29

J

J.B. Mattison, 2-519

Jackson, Charles T., 2-443

Jackson, John Hughlings, 1-21

Jacobi, Karl Wiegand Maximilian, 1-101

Jacobsen, Erik, 2-311

Jaffe, Jerome, 2-521

JAMA, *see* Journal of the American Medical Association (JAMA)

Jamison, Kay, 3-285

Janet, Pierre, 1-15, 1-16, 3-331

Jansen, Hans and Zacharias, 1-183

Janssen, Paul, 1-314, 1-316, 1-318, 1-319, 1-321, 1-358, 2-75–2-77, 2-79–2-82, 2-168, 3-24, 3-472, 3-789

Jaspers, Karl, 1-19, 1-20, *1-20*, 3-712, 3-715

jaundice, 1-52, 1-121, 1-127, 1-136, 1-340, 2-286, 2-511, 3-15

Jerne, Niels Kaj, 2-398

Johnson, Enid, 2-447

Jones, John, 2-452, 2-508

Jordan, Bertrand, 3-543

Journal of the American Medical Association (JAMA), 2-11, 2-520, 3-241, 3-453

Judge Joseph L. Tauro, 3-136

Judson, Walter E., 2-29

Jung, C., 2-534

Jung, Carl Gustav, 3-715

K

Köller, Carl, 2-445, 2-529

Kölliker, Rudolph Albert von, 1-187

Kühne, Friedrich Wilhelm, 1-190, 1-202

Kühne, Wilhelm Friedrich, 1-202

K-hole, *see* ketamine

Kahlbaum, Karl Ludwig, 3-327

Kahn, Robert E., 3-616

kairina, 1-130

kairolina, 1-130

Kalinowsky, Lothar B., 3-346

Kamin, Leon J., 1-401

Kane, H.H., 2-522

Kapha, *see* Ayurveda

Katast, *see* ketamine

Katz, Bernard, 1-205, 1-236

kava (Piper methysticum), 1-359

Keats, John, 2-439

Kefauver-Harris Amendment (1962), 2-81, 3-49

Kekulé, Friedrich A., 2-267

Kennedy, John F., 2-281, 3-496

kernicterus, 2-286

Kesey, Ken, 2-549, 3-128

Ketajet, *see* ketamine

Ketalar, *see* ketamine

ketamine, 1-305, 1-307, 1-405, 2-355, 2-486, **3-22**, 3-22, **3-23**, 3-23, **3-24**, 3-24, 3-26, 3-27, 3-216, 3-350, 3-642, 3-643
    antidepressant, 3-24
    K-hole, 3-24
    Katast, 3-24
    Ketajet, 3-24
    Ketalar, 3-24
    Ketanarkon, 3-24
    Ketanest, 3-24
    Ketavet, 3-24
    Kit Kat, 3-24

model of schizophrenia, 3-24
special K, 2-486, 3-24
Super Acid, 3-24
Super C, 3-24
Vetalar, 3-24
Ketanarkon, *see* ketamine
Ketanest, *see* ketamine
Ketavet, *see* ketamine
ketoconazole, 3-640
Khan, Hakim Ajmal, 2-30
khat, 1-133, 1-147, *see also* cathinone
Catha edulis, 3-796
kidney, 2-7, 2-275, 2-283, 2-532, 3-133
Killer Weed, *see* phencyclidine
kindling, 2-204, 3-348, 3-349, 3-664
King Charles III, 3-740
King Edward, 2-29
King Ferdinand VI, 3-740
King Hammurabi, 3-87, 3-123
King James I, 2-500
King Philip II, 2-464, 3-738
King Tutankhamen, 3-435
Kit Kat, *see* ketamine
Klaesi, Jakob, 2-273
Klein, Melanie, 1-21
Kline, Nathan, 1-22, 1-419, 2-10, 2-34, 3-367, 3-504
Kline, Nathan S., 2-32, 2-187
Koch, Robert, 2-338
Koepfli, Joseph, 2-29
Kola, 1-140, 1-146, 1-151–1-153
Kola nut, 1-153, 2-456
Kolb, Lawrence, 2-514
Kosterlitz, Hans W., 1-242, 2-422
Kraepelin, Emil, 1-xv, 1-11–1-13, 1-18, 1-21, 1-26, 2-6, 2-326, 2-328, 2-329, 2-332, 2-404, 3-228, 3-322, 3-327, 3-330, 3-712, 3-714, 3-721, 3-730, 3-743, 3-750
Krafft-Ebing, Richard von, 3-187
Kramer, 1-59, 2-435, 3-313, 3-315
Krause, Karl Friedrich, 3-741

Kretschmer, Ernst, 1-20
Kreuzelschreiber, 3-97
Kuhar, M.J., 1-171
Kuhn, Roland, 1-xiii, 1-22, 1-87, 1-336, 1-421, 2-12, 2-13, 2-111, 2-126, 2-127, 2-129, 2-135, 2-407, 3-11, 3-364–3-369, 3-504
Kuhn, T.S., 1-28

L

López-Ibor, Juan José, 2-37, 3-328, 3-715, 3-723, 3-731, 3-744, 3-745, 3-747, 3-766, 3-775, 3-800
L-acetylmethadone, *see* acetyl-methadone
L-deprenyl, *see* selegiline
Laënnec, René, 1-105
LAAM, *see* levacetylmethadol
Laborit, Henri Marie, 1-21, 1-308, 1-309, 1-420, 2-7, 2-35, 2-55, 2-56, 2-60–2-63, 2-65, 2-71, 2-225, 2-230, 2-407, 3-6, 3-9, 3-10, 3-215, 3-361, 3-362, 3-364, 3-368, 3-475, 3-790
labyrinth, 1-396, 3-408
lactation, 1-405
lactoferrin (LF), 1-151
lactucarium, 1-131, 1-146, 1-151
Lafora, Gonzalo Rodríguez, 3-712, 3-715, 3-722, 3-742, 3-744, 3-801
Laguna, Andrés, 1-61, 2-438, 2-492
Laing, Ronald David, 1-22
Lamalou, 1-141
Lamarck, Jean-Baptiste, 2-518
Lambert, Pierre A., 2-191
Lamiaceae, 2-466
Lamictal, *see* lamotrigine
lamotrigine, 1-334, 1-379, 2-197, 2-204–2-206, 2-211, 2-313, 3-336
Lamictal, 2-313

Lange, Carl, 2-364
Langley, John Newport, 1-153, 1-169, 1-205, 1-234
Lanzer, Ernst, 1-16
Largactil, *see* chlorpromazine (CPZ)
large intestine, 3-495
Lasègue, E. Charles, 1-6
Lasagna, Louis C., 3-375
Lassen, Niels, 2-82
laudanum, *see* opium
   ingredients, 2-507
   Sydenham's, 1-68, 1-124, 2-452
   tincture of opium, 2-4, 2-328, 2-414
Lavater, Johann Kaspar, 3-186
Lavedan, Antonio, 2-458
lavender, 2-361
Le Beau, 1-xxiv
Leary, Timothy, 2-537, 2-550, 2-551, 3-498
leech, 1-190
leeches, 1-42, 1-69, 2-331, 3-375, 3-439
Leeuwenhoek, Antoine van, 1-183, 1-186, 1-190
Lefort, P., 1-129
leg, 2-436
legal medicine, 3-791
Legrain, Paul Maurice, 1-9
Legrand du Saulle, 1-14
Lehmann, Heinz E., 2-8, 2-13, 2-35, 2-69–2-71, 2-129, 3-6, 3-8, 3-793
Lemaire, Charles, 2-534
Lemon balm, 2-455
Lempérière, Therese, 2-34
lens, 1-189, 1-190, 2-82, 2-441
Lenz, Fritz, 3-89, 3-97
leprosy, 2-447, 2-511, 3-429, 3-430
LeRoy, J.B., 3-343
lesion, 1-15, 1-293, 2-225, 2-341
leukocyte, 3-298, 3-299
Leuret, François, 1-7, 1-106
levacetylmethadol, 3-69
   LAAM, 2-308, 2-309
   levomethadyl acetate, 2-308

Levenstein, Eduard, 1-111
levetiracetam, 1-330, 2-210
Levine, Jerome, 2-537
levomepromazine, *see* methotrimeprazine
levomethadyl acetate, *see* levacetyl-methadol
levorphanol, 2-420
Lewin, Louis, 1-xxiii, 2-533, 3-491
Lewy Body dementia, 2-381, *see also* Parkinson's disease
Lewy, Fritz H., 3-714
Leyden, Ernst von, 1-118
LH, *see* luteinizing hormone
Li Shi Zhen, 1-66
Librium, *see* chlordiazepoxide
licarbazepine, 2-210
Liebermann, Carl, 2-58
Liebreich, Oscar, 1-110, 1-118, 1-305, 2-253, 2-254, 2-256, 2-266, 2-363
light-dark box test, 1-395
Lilly 110140, *see* fluoxetine
Lima, Almeida, 2-341
limbic system, 1-220, 2-222, 2-349, 3-504, 3-649, 3-664
Lindqvist, Margit, 2-45
linkage analysis, 1-288–1-290, 1-292, 1-293
Lipitor, *see* atorvastatin
liposome, 3-568, 3-570
liquid ecstasy, *see* γ-hydroxybutyric acid (GBH)
Lister, Joseph, 2-431
lithium, 1-ix, 1-xxiv, 1-129, 1-267, 1-361, 1-364, 1-376, 1-377, 1-379, 1-380, 1-382, 1-385, 1-418, 1-419, 1-444, 1-448, 1-451, 2-7, 2-181, 2-183–2-187, 2-189, 2-192–2-194, 2-197, 2-203, 2-204, 2-206, 2-207, 2-209, 2-311, 2-325, 2-363–2-365, 2-367, 3-3, 3-13, 3-14, 3-277, 3-278, 3-285, 3-310–3-312, 3-314, 3-316,

3-504, 3-512–3-514, 3-517, 3-518, 3-520, 3-523, 3-606, 3-625, 3-633, 3-755, 3-769, 3-798, 3-800
lithium carbonate, 2-7, 2-181, 2-183, 2-186, 2-187
lithium inhibition, 3-512
lithium salts, 1-xxvii, 1-21, 1-154, 1-418, 2-181, 2-184, 3-14, 3-327, 3-626
petalite, 2-7
lithium carbonate, *see* lithium
lithium inhibition, *see* lithium
lithium salts, *see* lithium
Liu, C.N., 1-174
liver, 1-44, 1-50, 1-184, 1-294, 1-359, 1-420, 2-110, 2-169, 2-193, 2-275, 2-283, 2-284, 2-312, 2-313, 2-528, 3-64, 3-69, 3-133, 3-641, 3-667, 3-732
liver colic, 1-132
liver failure, 2-561
acute, 3-69
Llorach, Pablo, 3-720
Llull, Ramon, 2-438, 2-491, 3-735
lobbying, 3-37, 3-241
lobotomy, 1-xxiv, 1-19, 1-21, 2-225, 2-343
chemical, 2-65, 3-6
local anesthetic, 1-112, 1-132, 1-148, 1-151, 1-529, 2-445, 2-456, 2-477, 3-198, 3-497
Locock, Charles, 1-328, 2-259, 2-261, 2-267
Loewenthal, H., 1-136
Loewi, Otto, 1-169, 1-205, 1-235, 2-14, 3-5, 3-593
lofepramine, 1-336, 2-135
Lombroso, Cesare, 1-10, *1-10*, 3-186–3-188, 3-206
Long, Crawford, 2-443
Long, Loren M., 1-333
Lophophora williamsii, *see* peyote

Lorente, Román Alberca, 3-715, 3-731
Lorenz, K., 1-226
Lorichius, Reinhardus, 1-xxiv
Los Avisos Sanitarios, 1-127
Lotmar, Fritz, 3-714
Louis XIV, 2-414, 2-439, 2-500
LSD, *see* lysergic acid diethylamide (LSD), *see* lysergic acid diethylamide, 3-237
LSD-25, *see* lysergic acid diethylamide (LSD)
LSD-25, *see* lysergic acid diethylamide (LSD)
Ludwig, Arnold M., 2-537
Lugaro, Ernesto, 1-206, 3-714, 3-756
lumbar, 1-442, 1-481, 1-488, 1-491, 1-494
Luminal, *see* phenobarbital
luminal sodium, 1-160
Lund, 1-240, 2-45
Lundbeck, 2-75, 2-82, 2-130
Lundy, John S., 2-278
Luneberg, 2-500
Lunesta, *see* zopiclone
lung, 1-284, 1-285, 1-449
lupus erythematosus, 3-67
lurasidone, 2-98
luteinizing hormone
LH, 2-63
LY-354740, *see* eglumegad
Lyman, Henry M., 2-443
lymphocyte, 2-390
lymphoma, 3-715
Lyrica, *see* pregabalin
lysergic acid, 2-462, 2-465, 2-484, 2-485, 2-545
lysergic acid diethylamide
LSD, 2-356
lysergic acid diethylamide (LSD), 1-xxiv, 1-162, 1-462, 1-463, 1-465, 1-480, 2-6, 2-15, 2-32, 2-96, 2-308, 2-311, 2-314, 2-348, 2-355, 2-447, 2-462–

2-464, 2-485, 2-535–2-537,
2-543, 2-545–2-547, **2-548**, 2-
548–2-552, 3-15, 3-54, 3-199,
3-210, 3-237, 3-505, 3-594,
3-762, 3-763
as a weapon, 3-237
Delysid, 2-535, 2-548–2-551
ergotherapy, 2-549
fathers of LSD|hyperpage, 2-550, 2-
551
LSD parties, 2-551
lysergide, 3-54
psychedelic therapy, 1-xxiv, 2-447,
2-536, 2-549
lysergide, *see* lysergic acid diethylamide
(LSD)

M

M'Meens, R.R., 2-519
M1, *see* methylone
Mühlethaler, K., 1-170
Müller, Charles, 1-3, *1-4*, 1-84
Müller, Johannes, 2-30, 2-31, 2-454
M-ECT, *see* maintenance ECT (M-ECT)
Ma Huang, *see* ephedra
Macbride, David, 2-333
Macht, David I., 1-xxv, 2-6
Maclean, Paul D., 3-414
MacLeod, Neil, 2-267
macromolecules, 3-582, 3-583
Maddox, Harold, 3-22
Madrid Declaration, 3-82, 3-88
Magendie, François, 1-110, 1-118
Magnan, Valentin, 1-9, 1-12, 3-187
magnesium sulfate, 1-159, 1-160
Magnus, Albertus, 2-359
Maier, Hans W., 2-275
Maimon, Moshe ben, 3-733
maintenance ECT (M-ECT), 3-354,
3-355
major depression, *see* major depressive
disorder
major depressive disorder

major depression, 1-245, 1-343,
1-356, 1-357, 1-421, 1-480,
1-483, 1-484, 1-486, 1-488,
1-490, 1-492, 2-156–2-158,
2-171, 2-173, 2-174, 2-176,
2-401, 2-402, 2-404, 2-405, 2-
408, 2-562, 3-83, 3-94, 3-131,
3-246, 3-292, 3-293, 3-313,
3-315, 3-331, 3-401, 3-447,
3-466, 3-512, 3-517, 3-518,
3-520, 3-639, 3-646, 3-647
recurrent depression, 2-7, 2-364, 3-
313
unipolar depression, 1-487, 2-160
malaria, 1-72, 1-141, 2-70, 2-338–2-340,
2-364, 2-406, 2-407, 2-447, 2-
494, 2-516, 3-374
Malarine, 1-146
malate dehydrogenase (MDH), 3-563
MALDI-TOF, 3-556, 3-557
MALDI-TOF-TOF, 3-556
malignant, 2-246, 2-434, 3-294
malleus, 1-59, 2-435
malonal, 1-151, 2-268
diethylmalonilurate, 1-151
malonyl urea, *see* barbituric acid
malonylurea, *see* barbituric acid
Malpighiaceae, 2-463, 3-797
Mandragora officinalis, *see* Mandrake
Mandragora officinarum, *see* Mandrake
mandragorine (mixture of atropine
and hyoscine), 2-434, *see also*
atropine
Mandrake, 1-42, 1-119, 2-3, 2-359,
2-361, 2-432, 2-434, 2-436,
2-438, 2-439, 2-447, 2-449,
2-506
Atropa mandragora, 2-3
Mandragora officinalis, 2-361
Mandragora officinarum, 2-447
root, 1-37, 2-438
mania, 1-xv, 1-5, 1-11, 1-40–1-42, 1-49,
1-51, 1-52, 1-65, 1-88–1-90,

1-93, 1-94, 1-109, 1-131, 1-134, 1-168, 1-262, 1-364, 1-418, 1-491, 2-4, 2-7, 2-181, 2-184–2-187, 2-193, 2-196, 2-197, 2-204–2-206, 2-208–2-211, 2-328, 2-329, 2-332, 2-336, 2-363, 2-364, 2-442, 2-448, 2-513, 2-519, 3-278, 3-285, 3-306, 3-310, 3-312, 3-336, 3-362, 3-438, 3-439, 3-474, 3-523, 3-526, 3-594, 3-735, 3-736, 3-738, 3-740, 3-741, 3-793

with delirium, 1-5

without delirium, 1-5, 1-6

manic agitation, 2-63, 2-65, 2-67, 3-362

Mann, Thomas, 3-286

Mao Tse-tung, 2-508

MAO-B, 1-339, 1-340, 1-357, 2-111, 2-112, 2-353

maprotiline, 1-339, 1-352, 1-357, 1-362, 2-135, 2-136, 2-172, 3-451, 3-459, 3-626, 3-769

Marín y Sancho, Francisco, 1-145

Marañón, Gregorio, 3-571, 3-711, 3-800

Marco Polo, 2-436

Mardones, Jorge, 3-801

Mariani, Angelo, 2-455, 2-527

Mariano, Don, 3-491

Marie, Pierre, 3-714

marijuana, see cannabis

Marinol, see tetrahydrocannabinol (THC)

Markingson, Dan, 3-249

Marks, Isaac, 3-13

marrow, 1-154, 1-329, 1-332, 3-568

Marsilid, see iproniazid

Martín-Santos, Luis, 3-716, 3-731

Martens, Lennart, 3-565

Martin, Joyce A., 2-537

Martin, William, 2-308

Marxow, Ernst Fleischl von, 2-477, 2-529

mass spectrometry (MS), 1-359, 1-362–1-365, 1-376, 1-377, 1-381, 1-385, 3-554, 3-556, 3-558, 3-559, 3-563, 3-564

mastication, 2-455, 2-476, 3-197

Matías, Ramón López, 3-741

matrix, 1-44, 1-229, 3-229, 3-547, 3-560

matrix-assisted laser desorption/ionization (MALDI), 3-556

Matteucci, Carlo, 1-186

Matthiessen, Augustus, 2-364

Mattioli, Pietro Andrea, 1-61, 2-517

Maudsley, Henry, 1-10, 2-326, 2-512

Maximilian de Crinis, 3-97, 3-100

mazindol, 3-67

McCririck, Pauline, 2-537

MDL-100907, see volinanserin

MDMA (methylenedioxymethamphetamine), **2-537**, 3-200

   Adam, 2-480

   Ecstasy, 2-355, 2-460, 2-480, 2-537, 2-538, 3-189, 3-200, 3-201, 3-206, 3-215

   XTC, 2-480

mead, 1-xxiii, 2-265, 2-490

mebanazine, 2-12, 2-107

meconarceine, 1-149

meconic acid, 1-149

   meconium, 1-124, 2-413

meconium, see meconic acid

medica, 2-256, 2-472, 2-492, 2-495, 2-506, 2-517, 3-347, 3-491

medical amphetamine, 2-349

MEDLINE, 1-376, 2-68, 3-35, 3-38, 3-114, 3-226, 3-619

Medrol, see methylprednisolone

medulla, 1-225, 1-467

Meehl, Paul E., 3-333

mefenorex, 3-67

   Anexate, 1-509

meiosis, 1-288

melancholy, 1-5, 1-6, 1-40, 1-41, 1-43, 1-48, 1-50–1-52, 1-97, 1-131,

1-132, 2-65, 2-182, 2-330, 2-335, 2-404, 2-511, 2-513, 2-517, 2-521, 2-527, 3-327, 3-331, 3-344, 3-731, 3-736, 3-738, 3-740

melanocyte, 3-769

melatonin, 1-490, 3-610, 3-647, 3-648

melitracen, 1-339

melitracene, 2-135

melitracene, *see* melitracen

memantine, 2-313, 2-355, 2-388, 2-389, 3-27, 3-643

Namenda, 2-313

membrane potential, 1-233, 1-262, 3-598, 3-600

memory disorders, 1-343, 3-669

Mendizábal, 3-718, 3-731, 3-741

Menelao, 3-494

meninges, 1-8, 1-105

meningitis, 1-107, 1-136, 3-63

meningoencephalitis, 2-391

Mennecke, Friedrich, 3-94, 3-100

menopause, 3-633

Menschenhülsen, Leere, 3-94

menstrual cycle, 3-467, 3-471

menstruation, 1-44, 1-108, 1-123, 3-467, 3-738

mental disease, 1-xxv, 1-27, 1-99, 1-101, 1-104, 1-106, 1-393, 2-55, 2-68, 2-69, 2-261, 2-406, 3-84, 3-295, 3-404

mental illness, 1-xiii, 1-xxvi, 1-xxix, 1-4–1-9, 1-11, 1-19, 1-21–1-23, 1-25–1-27, 1-35, 1-43, 1-45, 1-47, 1-48, 1-52, 1-53, 1-59, 1-75, 1-82, 1-86, 1-87, 1-90, 1-95–1-107, 1-109–1-112, 1-157, 1-462, 2-3, 2-10, 2-14, 2-17, 2-167, 2-225, 2-229, 2-341, 2-363, 2-495, 2-496, 2-505, 2-512, 2-518, 2-522, 2-537, 3-37, 3-42, 3-78, 3-80, 3-82, 3-88, 3-137, 3-158, 3-172, 3-173,

3-176, 3-227–3-229, 3-232, 3-245, 3-246, 3-249, 3-257, 3-278–3-281, 3-283–3-287, 3-291, 3-294–3-298, 3-300, 3-327, 3-328, 3-330, 3-331, 3-334, 3-335, 3-337, 3-375, 3-384, 3-399, 3-400, 3-406, 3-419, 3-705, 3-706, 3-708, 3-711, 3-718, 3-719, 3-721, 3-727, 3-730, 3-736, 3-750

mental retardation, 2-34, 2-523, 3-99, 3-293, 3-343, 3-419

meperidine, 1-316, 2-61, 2-420, 3-473–3-475

Dolatin, 3-475

Dolosal, 2-62–2-64

pethidine, 1-309, 1-316, 2-76, 2-77, 3-54

mephenesin, 1-162, 1-322, 2-11, 2-220–2-222

mephobarbital, *see* methylphenobarbital

meprobamate, 1-117, 1-162, 1-322, 1-323, 1-329, 1-377, 2-7, 2-10–2-13, 2-220, 2-222, 2-223, 2-225, 2-226, 2-229, 2-232, 2-363, 2-365, 2-407, 3-54, 3-140, 3-662, 3-755, 3-763

Equanil, 2-11, 2-222

Miltown, 2-11, 2-219, 2-222

Meratran, *see* pipradrol

mercaptopurine, 3-545

Merck, E., 2-266, 2-268

Mercy, E.E., 2-443

Mering, Josef Freiherr von, 2-268

Merritt, Houston, 1-328, 2-278

Mescalero Apaches, *see* American Indians

mescaline, 1-154, 1-159, 1-162, 1-304, 1-462, 2-6, 2-348, 2-355, 2-445, 2-447, 2-449, 2-464, 2-486, 2-533, 2-534, 2-537, 2-548, 2-550, 3-210, 3-491,

3-498

mesencephalon, 1-467, 1-528

Mesmer, Franz Anton, 1-67

messenger RNA (mRNA), 1-264, 1-281, 1-283, 1-296, 2-153, 3-512, 3-514, 3-517, 3-518, 3-521, 3-546–3-548, 3-550, 3-552, 3-553, 3-566, 3-569, 3-570, 3-635, 3-645

mesuximide, 1-333

meta-analysis, 1-427, 1-436, 1-437, 2-138, 2-172, 2-174, 2-175, 2-197, 2-205, 2-225, 2-310, 2-313, 2-314, 2-384, 3-230, 3-352, 3-386, 3-387, 3-455, 3-471, 3-472, 3-506, 3-507, 3-563

meta-chlorophenylpiperazine (mCPP), 2-370

metabolism, 1-158, 1-216, 1-228, 1-292–1-294, 1-322, 1-323, 1-337, 1-339–1-341, 1-358, 1-362, 1-363, 1-382–1-384, 1-386, 1-451, 1-466, 1-468, 1-481–1-483, 1-486–1-488, 1-490, 1-492–1-494, 2-60, 2-61, 2-67, 2-76, 2-130, 2-169, 2-221, 2-310, 2-382, 2-464, 2-537, 2-558, 3-9, 3-156, 3-216, 3-298, 3-349, 3-401, 3-467, 3-511, 3-561, 3-562, 3-570, 3-584, 3-585, 3-612, 3-628, 3-631, 3-635, 3-637, 3-774, 3-785

metachloral, 1-131

metapramine, 3-769

methadone, 2-76, 2-308–2-310, 2-314, 2-315, 2-420, 2-472, 2-476, 2-505, 2-510, 2-514, 2-563, 3-54, 3-69, 3-83, 3-196, 3-451
  addiction treatment, 2-308, 2-309, 2-314
  Dolophine, 2-308, 2-514

methaminodiazepoxide, see chlordiazepoxide

methamphetamine, 1-347, 2-308, 2-314, 2-349, 2-479, 2-480, 3-199, 3-526, 3-658
  methylamphetamine, 2-355, 2-480, 3-236

methaqualone, 1-334, 2-293

methergine, see methylergometrine

methohexital, 2-279, 2-286, 2-338, 3-350
  Brevital, 2-279

methotrimeprazine, 1-361, 3-473
  levomepromazine, 2-95

methoxytyramine, 2-17

methyl alcohol, 3-202

methyl-propyl-carbinol-urethane, 1-149, 1-158

methylal, see dimethoxymethane

methylamphetamine, see methamphetamine

methylation, 1-331, 1-462, 3-565, 3-566

methyldopa, 3-307

methylene blue, 1-147, 1-201, 1-307, 2-58, 2-126
  blue methylene, 1-151

methylergometrine
  methergine, 2-545
  methylergonovine, 2-545

methylergonovine, see methylergometrine

methylmorphinan, 2-416

methylol, 1-133

methylone
  M1, 2-386

methylphenidate, 1-347, 1-405, 2-84, 2-310, 2-350, 2-351, 2-480, 2-524
  Ritalin, 1-162, 2-310

methylphenobarbital
  mephobarbital, 2-277
  Prominal, 2-277

methylprednisolone
  Medrol, 1-146

methylsulfonal, 1-158, 2-4

methyprylon, 3-140

metoclopramide, 1-318, 3-472

metrazol, *see* pentylenetetrazol

metrorrhagia, 2-518

metyrapone, 3-640

Meyer, Adolf, 1-13, 3-322

Meyer, Ludwig, 1-7

mianserin, 1-339, 1-360, 2-136, 3-299, 3-453, 3-455, 3-626, 3-642, 3-644, 3-769

  Tolvin, 2-136

microarray, 1-292, 3-526, 3-527, 3-550, 3-551, 3-560, 3-566

  DNA array, 1-282, 1-283, 3-547, 3-550

  DNA microarray, 3-526, 3-527

microscopic anatomy, 1-183, 3-756

midbrain, 1-223, 1-491, 2-144, 2-220, 3-606

mifepristone, 3-640

migraine, 1-127, 1-135, 1-136, 1-138, 1-141, 1-145, 1-150, 1-153, 1-158, 2-58, 2-278, 2-354, 2-448, 2-472, 2-498, 2-511, 2-516, 2-519, 2-524, 2-544, 2-546, 3-63, 3-448, 3-454–3-456, 3-467, 3-474

milacemide, 3-657

Miller, Arthur, 3-496

Miller, Charles A., 1-333

milnacipran, 1-343, 2-168, 2-171–2-174

Milne-Edwards, Henri, 1-119

Miltown, *see* meprobamate

minaprine, 3-67

mind altering agents, 3-186

Minsky, Marvin, 1-170

Mira y López, Emilio, 3-712, 3-731, 3-801

Mirabilis jalapa, 1-103, 1-108

Mirandola, Giovanni Pico della, 1-58

mirtazapine, 1-357, 1-360, 2-168, 2-174–2-176, 3-455, 3-460, 3-467, 3-517

  Remeron, 2-174, 2-175

Mitchell, Silas Weir, 1-14, 2-534

mitochondria, 3-526

Mitscherlich, Carl Gustav, 1-110

moclobemide, 1-341, 1-357, 2-110, 2-112, 2-114, 2-115, 3-453

modafinil, 1-350, 2-314, 2-351

Mogadon, *see* nitrazepam

molecular biology, 1-xxv, 1-xxvii, 1-171, 1-179, 1-277–1-279, 1-281, 1-295, 1-437, 2-239, 2-387, 2-424, 2-425, 3-3, 3-411, 3-543, 3-631, 3-794, 3-802

Moles, E., 1-150

molindone, 1-319

Molloy, Bryan B., 2-144

Monardes, Nicolás, 2-445, 2-455, 2-499

Monase, *see* α-ethyltryptamine

Monitor de la Farmacia y de la Terapéutica, 1-141

monoamine oxidase inhibitor (MAOI), 1-ix, 1-335, 1-339–1-341, 1-356, 1-357, 1-423, 1-479, 1-490, 1-491, 2-12, 2-15–2-17, 2-44, 2-96, 2-105, 2-107–2-115, 2-125, 2-167, 2-168, 2-285, 2-353, 3-277, 3-278, 3-315, 3-331, 3-332, 3-354, 3-367, 3-460, 3-504, 3-606, 3-610, 3-612, 3-625, 3-626, 3-628, 3-636, 3-642, 3-644, 3-747, 3-763–3-765, 3-768–3-770, 3-773, 3-774, 3-790

monochlorimipramine, *see* clomipramine

monoclonal antibodies, 3-558, 3-785

Monroe, Alexander, 2-441

Monroe, Marilyn, 2-282, 3-495, 3-496

Montezuma II, 2-534

Monti, Jaime, 3-802

Montmartre, 3-498

Montserrat, Don Mariano de, 3-491

Mood Stabilizers, 1-xxvii, 1-208, 1-250, 1-375, 1-379, 1-415, 1-444, 1-445, 2-189, 2-204, 2-206, 2-207, 2-211, 3-245, 3-277, 3-312, 3-336, 3-447, 3-520, 3-525

Moor, H., 1-170

Moos, Rudolf H., 2-398

Moraceae, 3-797

moral treatment, 1-xvii, 1-8, 1-80, 1-83–1-89, 1-91, 1-92, 1-98–1-100, 1-102–1-104, 1-106–1-108, 1-112

Moreau de Tours, Jacques-Joseph, 1-xxiv, 1-105–1-107, 2-5, 2-484, 2-518, 2-521, 3-187, 3-492, 3-496, 3-789, 3-790

Morel, Bénédict Augustin, 1-8, 1-104, 1-107, 1-108, 3-187, 3-327, 3-742

Moreno y Maíz, Tomás, 2-527

Morison, Alexander, 2-333

Morning glory (Convolvulaceae), 2-465, 3-797

Morpheus, 2-416, 2-442, 2-472

morphine, 1-80, 1-103, 1-110–1-112, 1-118, 1-119, 1-124, 1-131, 1-132, 1-134, 1-137, 1-140, 1-151, 1-154–1-157, 1-303, 1-408–1-410, 2-3, 2-4, 2-76, 2-256, 2-266, 2-272, 2-274, 2-305, 2-306, 2-308, 2-328, 2-361, 2-362, 2-405, 2-415–2-417, 2-420, 2-425, 2-442, 2-445, 2-446, 2-449, 2-453, 2-472, 2-475, 2-477, 2-496, 2-505, 2-509, 2-510, 2-513–2-515, 2-519, 2-520, 2-529, 3-54, 3-188–3-190, 3-192, 3-193, 3-195, 3-198, 3-208, 3-235, 3-451, 3-474, 3-491–3-493, 3-497, 3-563, 3-771, 3-773
addiction, 1-111, 1-132, 1-137, 2-305, 2-348, 2-475, 2-509, 2-529, 3-83, 3-344
addiction clinics, 2-307
morphium, 2-416, 2-442
treatment of addiction, 1-112, 2-496

morphine dependence, 3-772

morphinomimetic, 2-365, 2-422

morphium, see morphine

Morris, Desmond, 3-413

mortalin, 3-563

Morton, William, 1-305, 2-442, 2-443

mosapramine, 1-311

mouth, 1-155, 1-158, 1-385, 1-421, 2-38, 2-159, 2-171, 2-174, 2-175, 2-258, 2-295, 2-328, 3-131, 3-345, 3-375, 3-376, 3-434, 3-497

movement disorders, 1-467–1-469

mRNA, see messenger RNA (mRNA)

MS, see mass spectrometry (MS)

Muira puama, 1-146

multiple sclerosis, 1-169, 2-524, 3-228, 3-461, 3-559

muscarine, 1-234, 1-235, 2-433

muscarinic receptor coupled G proteins, 3-512

muscazone, 2-449

muscimol, 1-507, 2-235, 2-449

muscle, 1-141, 1-155, 1-185, 1-190, 1-202, 1-284, 1-292, 1-322, 1-463, 2-11, 2-111, 2-113, 2-225, 2-233, 2-239, 2-278, 2-285, 2-338, 3-5, 3-476, 3-601, 3-607

muscle relaxant, 1-322, 1-323, 2-221, 2-239, 2-294, 2-296, 2-338, 2-447, 3-349, 3-447, 3-605

musk, 1-73, 1-97, 1-119, 1-129, 1-150

mutagenesis, 1-279

mutation, 1-xv, 1-283, 1-288, 1-290, 1-514, 2-425, 3-544, 3-550, 3-567

mutism, 2-337

mydriasis, 1-155, 1-316, 2-448

myelin, 3-596

myelitis, 1-136
myocardial infarction, 1-488, 3-455, 3-456
myocarditis, 1-152, 2-285
Myristica fragrans, see nutmeg
Myristicaceae, 2-463, 3-797
myristicin, 2-463
Myrtaceae, 3-797
myrtol, 1-146
Mysoline, see primidone

N

N,N-dimethyltryptamine, see dimethyl-tryptamine (DMT)
N-methyl-D-aspartate, see N-Methyl-D-aspartic acid (NMDA)
N-Methyl-D-aspartic acid (NMDA), 1-262, 1-292, 1-293, 1-330, 1-405, 1-406, 1-451, 2-98, 2-312, 2-355, 2-387, 2-388, 3-21–3-23, 3-25, 3-27, 3-460, 3-507–3-509, 3-560, 3-563, 3-609, 3-636, 3-642–3-645, 3-656–3-660, 3-667, 3-669
    N-methyl-D-aspartate, 1-292, 1-451, 2-98, 2-312, 2-355, 2-387, 3-21, 3-507, 3-609, 3-636
N-methylglycine, see sarcosine
nabilone, 2-521
    Cesamet, 2-521
Nagai, Nagayoshi, 2-479
Nalline, see nalorphine
nalmefene, 2-315
nalorphine, 2-308, 2-420, 2-514
    Nalline, 2-308
naloxone, 1-530, 2-308, 2-310, 2-315, 2-420, 2-422, 3-460, 3-499, 3-771, 3-773
naltrexone, 1-530, 1-531, 2-308, 2-311–2-314
    6-beta naltrexol metabolite, 2-312
Namenda, see memantine
Nansen, Fridtjof, 1-194

napelina, 1-146
narceine, 1-131, 1-149
narceine meconate, 1-146
narcolepsy, 1-350, 2-4, 2-111, 2-272, 2-351, 2-357, 2-523–2-525, 3-215, 3-461
Narcosan, see hexobarbital
narcotics, 1-68, 1-97, 1-103, 1-109, 1-111, 1-119, 1-120, 1-123, 1-124, 1-138, 1-139, 1-147, 1-150, 1-151, 2-308, 2-326, 2-495, 2-510, 2-524, 2-528, 3-54, 3-189, 3-197, 3-198, 3-209, 3-374, 3-491
Narcotine, see noscapine
natriuretic, 3-562
nature of paranoia, 1-11
Navale, Santé, 2-55
NDA, see New Drug Application (NDA)
NE, see norepinephrine
neck, 1-44, 2-331
Neckam, Alexander, 2-359
necrosis, 2-110, 3-69
nefazodone, 3-69, 3-128, 3-626
negative feedback, 1-222, 1-262, 1-483, 1-489, 3-640
Nembutal, see pentobarbital
nemifitide, 1-363
neoendorphins, 2-422
Neonal, see butobarbital
neonatal, 1-401, 2-315
neostigmine
    prostigmine, 3-349
nephentes, 2-499
nerve, 1-xxiii, 1-73, 1-74, 1-121, 1-132, 1-169, 1-186, 1-190–1-196, 1-198, 1-199, 1-201–1-207, 1-234, 1-235, 1-240, 1-259, 1-262, 1-264, 1-283, 1-481–1-483, 2-14, 2-34, 2-60, 2-68, 2-106, 2-110, 2-137, 2-144, 2-390, 2-397, 3-5, 3-351, 3-353, 3-355, 3-593, 3-594,

3-596, 3-598, 3-600, 3-608,
3-639, 3-715, 3-757, 3-764
nerve stimulants, 1-146
nervine, 1-154, 1-155
nervous accidents, 1-126, 1-145
nervous breakdowns, 1-137
nervous hypochondria, 1-151
nervous sedative, 1-147
nervous tonics, 1-147
netrin-G1, 3-563
neuralgia, 1-121, 1-133, 1-134, 1-151, 2-510, 2-519
    postherpetic, 3-448, 3-450, 3-451
neurasthenia, 1-14, 1-112, 1-136–1-138,
1-140, 1-141, 1-143–1-145,
1-148, 1-149, 1-151, 1-153,
2-477, 3-325
neurasthenic, 1-127, 1-137, 1-144,
1-147, 1-157
neurobiology, 1-xiv, 1-117, 1-167, 1-168,
1-170, 1-172, 1-250, 1-409,
1-531, 3-228, 3-390, 3-399,
3-414, 3-419, 3-640
neurochemistry, 1-170, 1-233, 1-240, 1-277, 3-5, 3-760
neurodyne, 1-146, 1-151
neuroglia, 1-191
neurokinin-3 (NK3) receptor, 3-659
neurolepsy, 2-68
neurolytic, 2-67
neuromuscular depressants, 1-130
neuromuscular junction, 1-194, 1-202,
1-205, 1-234
neuron, 1-168–1-170, 1-186, 1-191,
1-196, 1-198, 1-199, 1-201,
1-202, 1-206, 1-207, 1-221,
1-223, 1-224, 1-226, 1-241,
1-253, 1-254, 1-262, 1-264,
1-466, 1-483, 2-14, 2-15,
2-144, 2-150, 3-400, 3-461,
3-552, 3-593, 3-594, 3-596,
3-600, 3-601, 3-606, 3-610,
3-630, 3-645

neuron theory, 1-184, 1-191, 1-194,
1-195, 1-198, 1-199, 1-201,
1-202, 1-205–1-207, 1-234
neuropathic states, 1-153
neuroplegic, 2-56, 2-66, 2-67
neuroquinine, 3-658
neuroscience, 1-167, 1-196, 1-205,
1-250, 1-277, 1-359, 1-367,
1-527, 2-24, 2-161, 3-256,
3-284, 3-337, 3-414, 3-560,
3-566, 3-642, 3-756, 3-774
neurotoxic, 1-364, 2-390, 3-27, 3-636, 3-658
neurotransmitter, 1-168, 1-170, 1-174,
1-205, 1-235, 1-240, 1-242,
1-243, 1-249, 1-255, 1-259,
1-260, 1-268, 1-281, 1-286,
1-288, 1-319, 1-336, 1-367,
1-369, 1-405, 1-447, 1-449,
1-451, 1-460, 1-462, 1-471,
2-15, 2-45, 2-56, 2-142, 2-144,
2-150, 2-154, 2-156, 2-176,
2-206, 2-235, 2-312, 2-313,
2-316, 2-349, 2-350, 2-357,
2-371, 2-372, 2-382, 2-386,
2-406, 2-408, 3-5, 3-334,
3-461, 3-505, 3-509, 3-512,
3-514, 3-521, 3-527, 3-558,
3-561, 3-567, 3-594, 3-596,
3-628, 3-630, 3-640, 3-660,
3-662, 3-796
neutropenia, 3-61
New Drug Application (NDA), 3-53, 3-252
New York State Psychiatric Institute, 3-324, 3-346
Newton, Isaac, 2-449
nexus, 2-45, 3-407
nialamid, see nialamide
nialamide, 2-12, 2-17, 2-107, 2-109, 3-765, 3-790
    nialamid, 2-110
nickel bromide, 1-132

Nicolson, David, 3-187
Nicot, Jean, 2-499
Nicotiana, 2-498
nicotine, 1-119, 1-123, 1-234, 1-284, 1-406, 1-514, 2-386, 2-451, 2-498, 2-499, 2-501, 3-563
nicotinic acetylcholine receptor (cholinergic), 1-171
nicotinic acid, 1-349, 2-5
nicotinic acid diethylamide, see nikethamide
Niemann, Albert, 1-112, 1-119, 1-304, 2-348, 2-445, 2-455, 2-526, 3-198, 3-497
Nieto-Sampedro, 1-174
Nietzsche, Friedrich, 3-89
nightshade (Solanaceae), 1-124, 1-133, 2-266, 2-434, 2-439, 2-448, 3-491, 3-797
nikethamide, 1-160, 1-349, 3-344
    coramine, 2-545, 3-344
    nicotinic acid diethylamide, 2-545
nirvaina, 1-146
nisoxetine, 2-146
nitrazepam, 1-506, 2-233, 2-295, 2-297
    Mogadon, 1-506, 2-233
nitroglycerin, 1-129
    trinitrine, 1-146
nitrous oxide, 1-305, 2-440–2-443, 2-448, 2-449, 3-27, 3-491
Nitsche, Paul, 3-94, 3-100
Nixon, Richard, 2-550
NMDA antagonist, 2-388, 3-25, 3-27, 3-644
Noce, Robert H., 2-34
nociceptin, 1-286
    orphanin, 1-400
nocturnal agitation, 1-145
nocturnal enuresis, 2-524, 3-462, 3-464
nomifensine, 3-64, 3-127, 3-626, 3-645, 3-769, 3-772, 3-773
non-benzodiazepine anxiolytics, **2-245**, 2-293

noradrenaline, see norepinephrine
norcaine, see benzocaine
norclozapine, 2-93, 2-99, 3-654
    ACP-104, 3-654
    DMC, 2-93
norepinephrine, 1-171, 1-205, 1-235, 1-237, 1-238, 1-240, 1-241, 1-249, 1-262, 1-295, 1-314, 1-336, 1-340, 1-341, 1-343, 1-356, 1-421, 1-424, 1-462, 1-466–1-470, 1-484, 2-15, 2-44, 2-106, 2-142, 2-167, 2-247, 2-350, 3-451, 3-453–3-455, 3-459, 3-460, 3-463, 3-510, 3-511, 3-514, 3-596, 3-598, 3-610, 3-625, 3-626, 3-628, 3-630, 3-633, 3-648, 3-664, 3-762, 3-764, 3-765, 3-769, 3-770, 3-773
    NE, 1-356, 1-357, 1-367–1-369, 1-483, 1-484, 1-487–1-491, 1-494, 2-15–2-17, 2-106, 2-107, 2-111, 2-112, 2-142, 2-144, 2-146–2-148, 2-150, 2-152, 2-155, 2-167, 2-168, 2-171, 2-173, 2-174, 2-176, 3-596, 3-600, 3-659
    noradrenaline, 2-137
norepinephrine reuptake inhibitor (NRI), 1-343, 2-176, 2-347, 3-451, 3-457, 3-464, 3-517, 3-626, 3-631, 3-634, 3-773
norfluoxetine, see seproxetine
normetanephrine (NMN), 2-17
Normud, see zimelidine
norpseudoephedrine, 3-67
northern blot, 3-551
nortriptyline, 1-337, 1-357, 1-361, 1-381–1-383, 2-132, 2-137, 2-144, 3-451, 3-452, 3-455
    Allegron, 2-132
noscapine, 2-416
    Narcotine, 1-110, 1-119, 1-131

nostal, 1-160

Novocain, *see* procaine

nucleolus, 1-188, 1-190

nucleotide, 1-282, 1-384, 3-512, 3-544, 3-548, 3-561, 3-565, 3-582

nucleus, 1-187, 1-188, 1-190, 1-199, 1-216, 1-223, 1-268, 1-358, 1-447, 1-449, 1-491, 1-493, 1-511, 1-528, 1-530, 1-531, 2-7, 2-12, 2-154, 2-267, 2-311, 2-382, 2-462, 2-479, 2-545, 3-9, 3-564, 3-570, 3-645, 3-653, 3-656, 3-659, 3-773

Nuremberg Code, 3-90, 3-93, 3-101, 3-107, 3-127, 3-170

nutmeg, 2-463, 3-185

Myristica fragrans, 2-463

Nyswander, Marie E., 2-308, 2-514

O

O'Shaughnessy, William Brooke, 2-518

obese, 3-471

obesity, 1-347, 2-161, 2-350, 2-524, 3-300, 3-462, 3-471, 3-653, 3-796

obsessive-compulsive disorder, 1-ix, 1-343, 1-444, 2-133, 2-135, 2-159, 2-160, 2-248, 2-401, 3-12, 3-82, 3-315, 3-447, 3-466, 3-664, 3-775

ocaperidone, 3-649

octopamine, 3-610

Odyssey, 2-451, 2-472, 2-490, 2-516, 3-492

Ogle, W., 2-41

Okasha, Ahmed, 1-xxviii

olanzapine, 1-314, 1-358, 2-98, 2-158, 2-192, 2-193, 2-197, 3-133, 3-134, 3-218, 3-234, 3-308, 3-312, 3-472–3-475, 3-506, 3-509, 3-653, 3-658

olfactory, 1-255, 2-154, 3-526

olfactory bulb, 1-199, 3-653

oligodendrocyte, 3-527

Olmedioperebea sclerophylla, 3-797

ololiuqui, 2-447, 2-465, 2-534, 2-538

Rivea corymbosa, 2-465, 2-538

Oms y Garrigolas, Luis, 1-119

ondansetron, 2-313, 3-472, 3-665

open field test, 1-394, 1-395

ophthalmoplegia., 1-151

opioid peptides, 1-242, 1-400, 2-420, 2-422, 2-423

opipramol

opipramole, 2-135

opipramole, *see* opipramol

opium, 1-42, 1-49, 1-50, 1-62, 1-67, 1-68, 1-90, 1-103, 1-104, 1-108, 1-110, 1-119, 1-121, 1-125, 1-131, 1-137, 1-151, 1-155, 1-160, 1-167, 1-286, 1-303, 1-305, 1-528, 1-529, 2-3, 2-5, 2-6, 2-58, 2-220, 2-256, 2-260, 2-265, 2-266, 2-305, 2-326–2-329, 2-360–2-362, 2-413–2-419, 2-432, 2-434, 2-438, 2-439, 2-442, 2-446, 2-449, 2-451–2-453, 2-472–2-475, 2-483, 2-487, 2-495, 2-505–2-518, 2-522, 2-523, 2-532, 3-54, 3-189, 3-190, 3-192, 3-196, 3-198, 3-209, 3-211, 3-433, 3-435, 3-492, 3-662, *see also* laudanum

Confessions of an English Opium-Eater, 3-492

The Mysteries of Opium Reveal'd, 2-452, 2-508

Hague Convention of 1912, 3-198

International Opium Convention, 2-510, 3-193, 3-198

laudanum, 1-168, 2-3, 2-256, 2-328, 2-361, 2-362, 2-414, 2-432, 2-452, 2-472, 2-484, 2-507, 2-508, 2-513, 3-190, 3-492

opium dens, 3-192
opium extract, 1-94, 2-436
opium juice, 1-37
opium pills, 2-414
Permanent Central Opium Board, 3-209
Second International Opium Convention, 3-209
opium poppy (Papaver somniferum), 1-528, 2-256, 2-361, 2-413, 2-451, 3-189, 3-435, *see also* opium
Opium Wars, 2-415, 2-472, 2-508, 3-189, 3-190
First, 2-508
Second, 2-508
Treaty of Nanking, 2-415
optic, 1-186, 1-196, 3-615
oral, 1-218, 1-385, 1-483, 2-33, 2-80, 2-111, 2-133, 2-192, 2-278, 2-295, 2-297, 2-340, 2-348, 2-558, 3-131, 3-192, 3-374, 3-383, 3-432, 3-439, 3-602, 3-617
ORG-24448, *see* farampator
organ, 1-47, 1-74, 1-99, 1-110, 1-122, 1-167, 1-168, 1-243, 1-277, 1-278, 1-284, 2-495, 3-109, 3-110, 3-129, 3-158, 3-343, 3-404, 3-553, 3-554, 3-556, 3-565, 3-593, 3-607, 3-612
organ of Corti, 1-199
organelle, 3-554
organism, 1-40, 1-62, 1-72, 1-73, 1-102, 1-110, 1-118, 1-148, 1-187, 1-190, 1-193, 1-213–1-215, 1-217–1-220, 1-224, 1-225, 1-229, 1-278, 1-281, 2-3, 2-56, 2-61, 2-283, 2-284, 2-406, 3-215, 3-280, 3-546, 3-553, 3-570, 3-582
orlistat, 3-471
orphanin, *see* nociceptin

Orquitina Fumouze, 1-143
Orta, García de, 2-517
Orta, Garcia de, 2-27
ortal sodium, 1-160
Ortega y Gasset, José, 3-711, 3-731
Orthotimic, *see* chlorpromazine (CPZ)
Ortiz, Tomás, 2-445, 2-455
Osler, William, 2-222, 2-519
Osmond, Humphry, 1-462, 2-311, 2-447, 2-536
osmosis, 2-550
osmotic pressure, 1-218
overdose, 1-132, 1-345, 1-357, 1-377, 1-506, 2-113, 2-159, 2-220, 2-229, 2-233, 2-281, 2-282, 2-285, 2-349, 2-432, 2-434, 2-472, 2-508, 2-509, 2-524, 2-556, 2-558, 2-560, 3-64, 3-67, 3-121, 3-132, 3-218, 3-314, 3-457, 3-493, 3-499, 3-628
ovum, 3-404
oxalic acid, 3-48
oxazepam, 1-323, 1-506, 2-233, 3-217
Serax, 1-506
Seresta, 2-233
oxcarbazepine, 1-334, 2-196, 2-197, 2-204, 2-209, 2-210, 2-313, 2-367
Trileptal, 2-196
Trilteptal, 2-313
oxytocin, 1-221

P

Pöldinger, Walter, 1-384, 2-132, 2-133
p-chloro-phenylalanine, *see* fenclonine
pacemaker, 1-220, 1-229
Pagal-Ka-Dawa, 2-27
pagoclone, 3-664
pain, 1-xvii, 1-40, 1-41, 1-97, 1-111, 1-120, 1-121, 1-124, 1-131, 1-134, 1-139, 1-142, 1-149, 1-157–1-159, 1-287, 1-305,

1-316, 1-332, 1-343, 1-377, 1-416, 2-3, 2-136, 2-138, 2-176, 2-194, 2-207, 2-210, 2-247, 2-334, 2-361, 2-414, 2-423, 2-425, 2-431, 2-432, 2-436, 2-438, 2-439, 2-441–2-444, 2-447–2-449, 2-475, 2-476, 2-507, 2-510, 2-543, 3-66, 3-131, 3-229, 3-278, 3-284, 3-328, 3-373, 3-386, 3-395, 3-416–3-418, 3-433, 3-439, 3-447, 3-448, 3-450–3-457, 3-459–3-461, 3-465, 3-467, 3-473–3-476, 3-646, 3-731, 3-772, 3-773

pain management, 2-423, 3-457, 3-461

Palade, George Emil, 1-169, 1-206

palate, 2-258

Palay, Sanford Louis, 1-169, 1-206

Palfium, *see* dextromoramide

paliperidone, 3-649

    9-hydroxyrisperidone, 1-364

pancreatitis, 2-193

panic disorder, 2-160, 2-161, 2-247, 2-248, 2-370, 2-401, 2-562, 3-82, 3-144, 3-217, 3-327, 3-523, 3-664

Papaver somniferum, *see* opium poppy (Papaver somniferum)

Papaveraceae, 1-154

papaverine, 1-131, 1-147, 1-160, 2-416

para-chloroamphetamine (PCA), 2-144, 2-150

Paraire, Jean, 1-309, 2-63

paraldehyde, 1-110, 1-127, 1-131–1-133, 1-140, 1-149, 1-151, 1-157, 1-352, 2-4, 2-220, 2-229, 2-265, 2-267, 2-276, 2-305, 2-329, 2-363, 2-512, 2-555, 3-491

paralyses, 1-127

paralysis, 1-8, 1-40, 1-65, 1-74, 1-105, 1-123, 1-136, 1-139–1-141, 1-155, 1-158, 1-201, 2-5, 2-220,

2-221, 2-334, 2-338, 2-339, 2-342, 2-406, 2-448, 2-501, 3-135, 3-202, 3-280, 3-332, 3-349, 3-607, 3-711, 3-740

paranoia, 1-5, 1-16, 1-19, 1-530, 2-357, 3-64, 3-65, 3-284, 3-749

parasympathetic, 1-234, 1-235, 2-14, 3-596

parathyroid hormone, 1-160

Parennin, Dominique, 1-66

paresis, 1-74

pargyline, 1-340, 2-112, 3-767

Parke-Davis Laboratories, 1-160, 1-161, 1-328, 1-333, 2-271, 2-519, 2-529, 2-533, 3-4, 3-22, 3-24

Parkinson's disease, 1-160, 1-169, 1-241, 1-263, 1-340, 1-358, 1-421, 1-466–1-468, 1-471, 1-493, 2-45, 2-105, 2-381, 3-228, 3-300, 3-563, 3-564, 3-604, 3-611

Parlodel, *see* bromocriptine

paroxetine, 1-341, 1-343, 1-356, 1-361, 2-141, 2-148, 2-157, 2-158, 2-168, 2-174, 2-175, 2-197, 3-131, 3-132, 3-246, 3-401, 3-453, 3-455, 3-464, 3-468, 3-645, 3-647, 3-668

Passiflora incarnata, 2-361

Pasteur, Louis, 2-492, 2-544

patch-clamp, 1-172

patent medicine, 2-305, 3-278

pathogenic, 1-16, 1-292, 1-293, 1-399, 1-486, 1-488, 3-327, 3-706

Patin, Guy, 2-439

Paullinia cupana, 2-456, 2-458, 3-796

Pavlov, 1-219, 1-393, 1-394, 2-276

Pavlov, I.P., 1-213

PCE, *see* eticyclidine

PCP, *see* phencyclidine

PCR, *see* polymerase chain reaction (PCR)

Peace, *see* phencyclidine

pellotine, 1-146, 1-154

Pemberton, John, 1-119
pemoline, 3-69
Pen Tsao Ching, 2-516
penicillin, 2-5, 2-11, 2-220, 2-339, 2-535, 3-4, 3-5, 3-280
Pentagastrin, 1-221, 1-226
Pental, 1-134, 1-149
pentapeptides, 2-421
pentazocine, 2-308, 2-420, 3-54, 3-645
pentetrazol, *see* pentylenetetrazol
pentobarbital, 1-160, 1-307, 1-506, 2-272, 2-278, 2-279, 2-281, 2-282, 2-285, 3-495
    Nembutal, 1-506, 2-272
pentotal, 1-160
Pentothal, *see* thiopental
pentylenetetrazol, 1-511, 2-5, 2-221, 2-239, 2-336, 3-344
    Cardiazol, 1-19, 2-125, 2-276, 2-306, 2-336, 3-344, 3-346, 3-347
    metrazol, 1-160, 2-306
    pentetrazol, 1-349
    PTZ, 1-511, 1-512
pepsin, 1-138
peptic ulcer, 2-398
Percival, Thomas, 3-87, 3-126
Pereira, Alfonso Arteaga, 1-159
Pereira, Gómez, 3-708, 3-709
peripheral nervous system (PNS), 1-142, 1-205, 1-215, 3-5, 3-368, 3-594–3-596, 3-601
peristalsis, 2-67
Permanent Central Opium Board, *see* opium
pernocton, 2-278
pernoston, 1-160
Peronine, *see* benzylmorphine
pertofrane, 3-12
PET, *see* positron emission tomography (PET)
Petersen, Paul Viggo, 2-82
pethidine, *see* meperidine

Peto, Richard, 3-240
Peyocactin, *see* hordenine
peyote, 1-159, 1-162, 1-303, 2-445, 2-449, 2-451, 2-464, 2-486, 2-534, 3-185, *see also* mescaline
    Lophophora williamsii, 1-304, 2-464, 2-533, 2-534
    teonanácatl, 1-304, 2-447, 2-464
peyote buttons, 2-534
peyote cactus, 2-486
phanodorm, 1-158, 1-160
phantastica, 1-162, 2-534, 3-491
pharmaceutical industry, 1-28, 1-111, 1-112, 1-117, 1-128, 1-376, 2-3, 2-41, 2-132, 2-135, 2-196, 2-347, 2-544, 3-3, 3-4, 3-21, 3-22, 3-35–3-37, 3-39, 3-41, 3-42, 3-110, 3-122, 3-137, 3-140–3-145, 3-225–3-227, 3-238–3-242, 3-244, 3-245, 3-247–3-249, 3-251, 3-253, 3-254, 3-256, 3-258, 3-278, 3-281, 3-284, 3-581, 3-587, 3-594, 3-633, 3-647, 3-794
pharmacophore, 1-328, 2-82, 3-27, 3-583
pharmacovigilance, 1-385, 3-48, 3-49, 3-52, 3-55, 3-57, 3-68, 3-141
Pharmacovigilance Risk Assessment Committee (PRAC), 3-53
phenacetine, 1-135, 1-151
phenanthrene, 2-416
phenbenzamine, 1-307, 2-56
phencyclidine, 1-405, 2-98, 2-355, 2-356, 3-22, 3-23, 3-26, 3-27, 3-507, 3-643, 3-656, 3-658
    Angel Dust, 2-355, 3-22, 3-507
    Dust, 1-136, 2-525, 3-22
    Elephant, 3-22
    Embalming Fluid, 3-22
    Hog, 3-22
    Killer Weed, 3-22
    model of schizophrenia, 3-23,

3-518

PCP, 1-404–1-406, 2-355, 3-22, 3-24–3-27, 3-507, 3-508

Peace, 1-162, 1-163, 3-22

Rocket Fuel, 3-22

Sernyl, 3-22

Sernylan, 3-22

Super Weed, 3-22

wet, 1-122, 2-334, 2-364, 3-463

phendimetrazine, 3-67

phenelzine, 1-341, 2-12, 2-107–2-110, 2-114, 2-310, 3-315, 3-327, 3-332, 3-350, 3-765

Phenergan, *see* promethazine

pheniprazine, 2-12, 2-107, 2-110, 3-765

phenmetrazine, 2-349, 3-67

phenobarbital, 1-150, 1-160, 1-328, 1-331, 1-378, 1-506, 2-4, 2-191, 2-209, 2-261, 2-270, 2-271, 2-276–2-279, 2-281, 2-283–2-286, 2-363, 3-68

Luminal, 1-150, 1-156, 1-158, 1-160, 1-328, 1-506, 2-270, 2-273, 2-277

phenobarbitone, 1-352, 2-277

phenobarbitone, *see* phenobarbital

phenothiazine, 1-162, 1-307–1-309, 1-311, 1-316, 1-319, 1-358, 2-7, 2-9, 2-58, 2-60, 2-82, 2-125–2-127, 2-365, 3-9, 3-11, 3-127, 3-130, 3-361, 3-362, 3-365, 3-368

phenothiazine derivatives, 1-357, 3-6

phenothiazines, 1-319, 1-321, 1-326, 1-358, 1-377, 2-7–2-10, 2-16, 2-23, 2-38, 2-41, 2-58, 2-93, 2-126, 2-185, 2-223, 2-308, 2-454, 3-9, 3-286, 3-299, 3-361, 3-362, 3-473, 3-772

phenoxybenzamine, 3-773

phenoxyphenylpropylamine, 2-146, 2-147

phensuximide, 1-333

phentermine, 2-350, 3-67

phentolamine, 3-764, 3-772

phenyl methyl acetone, 1-127

phenyl-isopropyl-amine, 2-479

phenylethylmalonamide (PEMA), 2-278

phenylpiperazines, 2-370

phenylurethane, 1-139

phenytoin, 1-328, 1-330, 1-331, 1-334, 1-349, 1-377, 2-209, 2-261, 2-278, 2-367, 3-667

diphenylhydantoin, 1-154, 3-384

diphenylhydantoin sodium, 1-161

pheochromocytoma, 1-283

phobic disorders, 2-315

phosphodiesterase inhibitors, 3-637

phosphoinositol 4,5-bisphosphate (PIP$_2$), 1-259, 3-598

phosphorus, 1-143, 1-147, 1-377, 1-447

phosphorylation, 1-250, 1-252, 1-253, 1-265, 1-267, 1-285, 3-509, 3-513, 3-517, 3-518, 3-553, 3-570, 3-571, 3-630, 3-631, 3-633, 3-634

physiology, 1-xxviii, 1-7, 1-21, 1-64, 1-117, 1-154, 1-168, 1-169, 1-172, 1-174, 1-185, 1-186, 1-190, 1-201, 1-203–1-205, 1-216, 1-219, 1-235–1-237, 1-240, 1-242, 1-252, 1-286, 1-287, 1-394, 1-434, 2-44, 2-55, 2-61, 2-137, 2-160, 2-184, 2-339, 2-343, 3-5, 3-280, 3-411, 3-415, 3-466, 3-504, 3-553, 3-569, 3-593–3-595, 3-601, 3-715, 3-756–3-758, 3-760, 3-761, 3-786, 3-787

physostigmine, 2-382, 3-218

phytotherapy, 1-359

Pi y Molist, Emilio, 3-718, 3-741

pia mater, 1-185

Pichot, Pierre, 1-xxiv, 3-327

picrotoxin, 1-129, 1-511, 3-604

pilocarpine, 1-146, 1-234, 2-307

pimavanserin, 3-652, 3-653
Pinel, Philippe, 1-3, *1-4*, 1-5, *1-5*, 1-6,
　　　1-8, 1-84–1-97, 1-105, 1-106,
　　　1-113, 2-326–2-328, 2-331,
　　　2-332, 2-343, 3-187, 3-321,
　　　3-322, 3-381, 3-717, 3-731,
　　　3-741, 3-790
pipamperone, 1-362, 2-81
pipradrol, 1-162
　　　Meratran, 1-162, 2-219
Piquer, Andrés, 3-735, 3-740
piracetam, 1-330, 3-644
piramidon, 1-146
pirenzepine, 3-465
piribedil, 3-773
Piscidia, 1-139, 1-147
Piscidia erythrina, 1-129, 1-134, 1-149
Pitta, *see* Ayurveda
pituitary gland, 1-484
pivaloyl-benzylhydrazine, 3-765
Pizarro, Francisco, 2-477, 2-525
placebo, 1-xvii, 1-xxviii, 1-369, 1-383,
　　　1-415, 1-416, 1-429, 1-446, 1-
　　　447, 2-7, 2-8, 2-13, 2-35, 2-85,
　　　2-108, 2-109, 2-112, 2-115,
　　　2-156–2-160, 2-170–2-176,
　　　2-185–2-187, 2-192, 2-194,
　　　2-197, 2-203–2-211, 2-225,
　　　2-247, 2-248, 2-297–2-299,
　　　2-311, 2-313–2-315, 2-367,
　　　2-370, 2-384, 2-388, 2-391,
　　　2-522, 2-557, 2-562, 3-14, 3-
　　　65, 3-81, 3-105, 3-112, 3-113,
　　　3-128, 3-131, 3-165, 3-176,
　　　3-217, 3-234, 3-252, 3-255,
　　　3-281, 3-305–3-311, 3-313–
　　　3-315, 3-350, 3-371–3-375,
　　　3-383–3-390, 3-450–3-457,
　　　3-462–3-468, 3-471–3-474,
　　　3-476, 3-509, 3-644, 3-647,
　　　3-649, 3-657, 3-658, 3-660,
　　　3-661
placenta, 2-283, 3-404

plague, 1-62, 2-415, 2-485, 2-499, 2-507,
　　　3-47
plasma, 1-254, 1-259, 1-262, 1-264,
　　　1-359, 1-363, 1-364, 1-375–
　　　1-378, 1-380–1-383, 1-385,
　　　1-386, 1-472, 1-481, 1-483,
　　　1-488–1-490, 1-492, 2-169,
　　　2-185, 2-209, 2-299, 3-453,
　　　3-456, 3-462, 3-464, 3-467,
　　　3-561, 3-640, 3-645–3-647,
　　　3-666, 3-769
platelets, 1-466, 1-481, 1-490, 2-158
Plato, 1-35–1-38, 1-43, 1-46, 1-184,
　　　3-379, 3-395, 3-736
Platter, Felix, 2-360
Plessis, Armand Jean du, 1-59
Pletscher, Alfred, 2-44
pleurisy, 1-143
plexus, 1-121
Plumier, Charles, 2-28
pneumonia, 2-4, 2-448, 2-532, 3-8, 3-97,
　　　3-235
Poe, Edgar Allan, 3-492
Pollack, Benjamin, 2-42
polymerase chain reaction (PCR),
　　　1-171, 1-278, 1-384, 3-526,
　　　3-546, 3-551, 3-566, 3-600
polymorphism, 1-288, 1-295, 1-386,
　　　1-485, 3-418, 3-507, 3-511,
　　　3-512, 3-514, 3-520, 3-544,
　　　3-550, 3-567
　　　genetic, 2-169
　　　restriction fragment length, 3-550
polyneuropathies, 2-494, 3-452, 3-454
polypeptide, 3-562, 3-610
Pomme, Pierre, 1-73
ponezumab, 2-391
Pope Leon XIII, 2-456, 2-478, 2-527
poppy (Papaveroideae), 1-xxiii, 1-119,
　　　1-131, 2-3, 2-359, 2-360,
　　　2-413, 2-415, 2-432, 2-436,
　　　2-438, 2-439, 2-446, 2-449,
　　　2-451, 2-472, 3-189, 3-190,

3-209, 3-435, 3-492, *see also*
    opium
    black poppy, 1-131
    common poppy, 1-131
    garden poppy, 1-131
    white poppy, 1-131
porphyria, 2-285
porphyrinuria, 1-158
Porsolt, Roger D., 1-176
positron emission tomography (PET),
        1-174, 1-242, 1-352, 1-368–
        1-370, 1-448–1-451, 1-483,
        1-484, 1-492, 1-493, 2-98,
        3-349, 3-505, 3-600, 3-638,
        3-652
post-flu neurasthenias, 1-153
postoperative nausea and vomiting, 3-
        472
posttraumatic stress disorder (PTSD), 1-
        253, 2-161, 2-401, 3-664, 3-667
potassium pump, 1-262
Potter, D.D., 1-170
Praag, Herman van, 2-137
Pravaz, Gabriel, 2-442
Pravdivtzev, V.A., 1-227
precocious dementia, *see* schizophrenia
pregabalin, 2-209, 2-210, 2-313, 3-666
    Lyrica, 2-313
pregnancy, 1-158, 1-269, 2-315, 2-404,
        2-510, 2-562, 3-110, 3-335
pregnenolone, 3-665, 3-666
Preiswerk, Ernst, 2-272
pressor effects of amphetamine, 2-348
priapism, 1-108
Prichard, James Cowles, 3-187
Priestley, Joseph, 2-440
primidone, 1-331, 2-278, 2-286
    Mysoline, 2-278
pro-opiomelanocortin, 2-422
procaine, 2-456
    beginning of Modern Anesthesiol-
        ogy|hyperpage, 2-456
    Novocain, 2-445

prodynorphin, 2-422
    derivatives, 2-422
Prohibition, *see* Volstead Act (1919)
prolactin, 1-314, 1-484, 1-492, 1-493, 2-
        96, 2-399, 3-467, 3-509, 3-652,
        3-656, 3-771, 3-775
promazine, 2-9, 2-133, 3-11, 3-361,
        3-473, 3-475
promethazine, 1-308, 1-309, 1-336,
        1-357, 2-7, 2-58, 2-60, 2-82,
        2-127, 2-219, 2-229, 3-361,
        3-362, 3-473, 3-475, 3-762
    3277 RP, 2-58, 2-59
    Phenergan, 2-58–2-61, 3-762
Prominal, *see* methylphenobarbital
Prondol, *see* iprindole
propanediol, 1-322, 2-7, 2-11, 2-221
properties, and convulsive ergotism, 2-
        543
propionate, *see* diethylketone
propiophenone, 1-316, 2-76
propizepine, 2-135
propofol, 2-279, 3-350
Proponal, *see* propylbarbital
propoxyphene, 2-511
propranolol, 3-307, 3-772
propylamine, 1-130
propylbarbital
    dipropylbarbituric acid, 1-156
    Proponal, 1-151, 1-156
propylhexedrine, 3-67
prostaglandin, 3-646
prostate, 3-456
prosthesis, 3-131
prostigmine, *see* neostigmine
protein binding, 3-570
protein folding, 3-561
proteomic, 1-xxvii, 1-xxviii, 1-283,
        3-527, 3-553, 3-554, 3-559,
        3-560, 3-562–3-565
Prothiaden, *see* dosulepin
proton, 1-335, 1-447, 3-464
protoplasm, 1-190, 1-196

protoxide of nitrogen, 1-129
protriptyline, 1-337, 1-357, 2-132
    Concordin, 2-132
    Vivactil, 2-132
Prozac, see fluoxetine
pseudohypericin, 1-364–1-366
psilocin, 1-304, 2-464
psilocybin, 1-304, 1-471, 2-348, 2-356,
    2-447, 2-537, 2-538, 3-499
psoriasis, 3-466
psychedelic therapy, see lysergic acid di-
    ethylamide (LSD)
psychiatric, 3-234–3-237
psychiatric disease, 1-245, 3-16, 3-389
psychic disease, 1-35
PsychInfo, 3-35
psychoanaleptic, 1-118, 3-795, 3-796
psychoanalysis, 1-xxiv, 1-14, 1-15,
    1-17–1-19, 1-21, 1-25, 1-26,
    1-28, 1-117, 2-230, 2-240,
    2-447, 2-477, 3-228, 3-245,
    3-322, 3-327, 3-383, 3-384,
    3-398, 3-399, 3-522, 3-711,
    3-712, 3-714–3-716, 3-723,
    3-745, 3-747, 3-791
psychodysleptic, 1-118, 2-464, 2-505, 3-
    497, 3-796
psycholepsy, 2-67
psycholeptic, 1-118, 2-13, 3-795, 3-796
psychological tension, 1-16, 2-67
psychomotor agitation, 2-79, 2-364
psychopathology, 1-14–1-17, 1-19–1-21,
    1-393, 1-394, 1-496, 2-97,
    2-187, 2-399, 2-560, 3-176,
    3-321, 3-326, 3-335, 3-336,
    3-363, 3-413, 3-415–3-417,
    3-705, 3-715, 3-727, 3-729,
    3-741, 3-744, 3-748–3-750
Psychopharmacologic Drugs Advisory
    Committee, see Food and
    Drug Administration (FDA)
psychoses, 1-12, 1-13, 1-18, 1-20, 1-25,
    1-162, 1-318, 1-480, 2-5,
    2-70, 2-71, 2-88, 2-105, 2-109,
    2-219, 2-220, 2-223, 2-338,
    2-402, 2-405, 2-496, 2-513,
    2-530, 2-534, 2-535, 3-132,
    3-205, 3-277, 3-286, 3-447,
    3-653, 3-750, 3-761
psychosomatic, 1-21, 2-398, 3-303,
    3-315, 3-316, 3-385, 3-447,
    3-464, 3-712, 3-715–3-717
psychotherapy, 1-xxviii, 1-14, 1-19,
    1-26, 1-102, 1-117, 1-162,
    1-436, 1-479, 2-37, 2-281,
    2-308, 2-348, 2-356, 2-481,
    2-535, 2-537, 3-110, 3-258,
    3-303, 3-305, 3-313, 3-373,
    3-382, 3-383, 3-395, 3-396,
    3-398, 3-399, 3-401–3-404,
    3-705, 3-710, 3-711, 3-715,
    3-738
psychotic, 1-ix, 1-xxiv, 1-17, 1-21, 1-309,
    1-319, 1-358, 1-403–1-406,
    1-451, 1-480, 2-17, 2-35, 2-37,
    2-41, 2-42, 2-81, 2-109, 2-126,
    2-181, 2-219, 2-222, 2-223,
    2-225, 2-230, 2-231, 2-240,
    2-273, 2-276, 2-283, 2-326,
    2-336, 2-340, 2-350, 2-370,
    2-384, 2-402, 2-405, 2-406,
    2-485, 2-521, 2-549, 3-15,
    3-67, 3-80, 3-82, 3-122, 3-127,
    3-134, 3-198, 3-231, 3-249,
    3-278, 3-279, 3-300, 3-322,
    3-333, 3-334, 3-351, 3-373,
    3-385, 3-447, 3-474, 3-499,
    3-504, 3-507, 3-522, 3-526,
    3-612, 3-652–3-654, 3-660,
    3-723
psychotic disorders, 1-178, 1-286, 1-
    401, 2-24, 2-26, 2-340, 2-348,
    2-549, 3-132, 3-293, 3-325,
    3-525, 3-654
psychotonic, 1-118
psychotropic drugs, 1-ix, 1-xxiv–1-

xxviii, 1-207, 1-351, 1-352,
1-359–1-363, 1-367–1-370,
1-375–1-377, 1-382, 1-384,
1-385, 1-415, 1-423, 1-424,
1-441, 1-448–1-450, 1-480,
2-6, 2-13–2-17, 2-38, 2-44,
2-46, 2-55, 2-167–2-169,
2-359, 2-409, 3-5, 3-47, 3-48,
3-54, 3-55, 3-58, 3-122, 3-123,
3-127, 3-128, 3-130, 3-136,
3-138, 3-140, 3-189, 3-208,
3-218, 3-225, 3-226, 3-228,
3-232, 3-234, 3-236, 3-238,
3-247, 3-251, 3-257, 3-258,
3-277, 3-286, 3-293, 3-298,
3-300, 3-308, 3-315, 3-369,
3-400, 3-403, 3-447, 3-448,
3-499, 3-610, 3-625, 3-760,
3-766, 3-767, 3-772, 3-774,
3-793, 3-798

PTZ, *see* pentylenetetrazol

puberty, 3-633

Pujadas, Antonio, 3-719

pulmonary, 1-105, 1-122, 1-151, 1-345, 2-475

pupil, 1-122, 1-124, 1-234, 2-79, 2-448

Purcell, Edgard M., 1-174

Pure Food and Drug Act (1906), 1-417, 2-528, 3-192, 3-198

Purkinje, Johannes Evangelist, 1-187

Pussin, Jean Baptiste, 1-3, 1-84, 1-92

pyramidol, 1-151

pyridine, 1-326, 1-331, 1-349, 1-512, 2-295, 3-655

pyridoxine (vitamin B6), 1-506

pyrithyldione, 3-67

pyrrolidone, 1-349, 3-644

Pythagoras, 2-438

Q

Qianlong, 1-66

quadriplegia, 3-603

Queen Victoria, 2-259, 2-444, 2-461, 2-518

quetiapine, 1-314, 1-358, 2-98, 2-193, 2-197, 3-218, 3-308, 3-474, 3-506

quietol, 1-151, 1-152

quinine, 1-66, 1-72, 1-90, 1-97, 1-110, 1-111, 1-121, 1-130, 1-146, 1-147, 1-150, 1-151, 1-159, 2-6, 2-260, 2-305, 2-306, 2-329, 2-330, 2-339, 3-374

quinochloral, 1-147

quinoline, 1-130

R

R 1625, *see* haloperidol

Rüdin, Ernst, 3-89

rabies, 2-325, 2-501, 3-570, 3-714

radioimmunoassay (RIA), 1-361, 1-362, 1-381, 1-382

radioligand, 1-xxvi, 1-171, 1-238, 1-242, 1-369, 1-370, 1-451, 2-150, 2-152, 2-235, 3-586, 3-600

Ramón Sarró, 2-37, 3-347, 3-711, 3-715, 3-716, 3-731, 3-745, 3-766, 3-800

Rameau, 1-81, 1-82

Rameses II, 3-432

Randall, Lowell, 1-322, 2-231, 3-504

randomized clinical trial, 1-428, 2-7, 2-35, 2-40, 2-110, 2-133, 2-138, 2-157, 2-158, 2-171, 2-173, 2-175, 2-176, 2-192, 2-205, 2-207, 2-209, 2-313, 2-384, 2-391, 3-13, 3-180, 3-217, 3-230, 3-249, 3-258, 3-278, 3-281, 3-307, 3-312, 3-352, 3-450, 3-456, 3-468, 3-509, 3-644, 3-647

ranitidine, 3-465

raphe, 1-450, 1-484, 1-485, 1-495, 2-144, 2-153, 3-664

Rathbun, Robert, 2-144

Rauwolf, Leonhard, 2-453

Rauwolfia serpentina, 1-162, 1-307, 1-460, 2-10, 2-15, 2-23, 2-24, 2-27–2-35, 2-38, 2-46, 2-453, 2-454, 3-762
    alkaloid, 2-126, 2-136
    sarpagandha, 2-24, 2-27
    Siledin, 2-33
    snakeroot, 2-27
Raymond-Hamet, M., 2-29
reboxetine, 1-343, 1-360, 3-457, 3-459, 3-464, 3-633, 3-634, 3-644, 3-646
receptor, 1-xxv, 1-171, 1-174, 1-196, 1-234, 1-236, 1-238, 1-241–1-243, 1-245, 1-257, 1-260, 1-262–1-264, 1-268, 1-280, 1-281, 1-284–1-287, 1-292, 1-294, 1-295, 1-311, 1-319, 1-330, 1-343, 1-358, 1-369, 1-379, 1-396, 1-399, 1-405, 1-406, 1-449–1-451, 1-471, 1-472, 1-481–1-493, 1-495, 1-506, 1-511, 1-512, 1-514, 2-45, 2-82, 2-85, 2-96–2-99, 2-142, 2-144, 2-150, 2-153, 2-154, 2-156, 2-158, 2-235–2-239, 2-245–2-247, 2-249, 2-293, 2-296, 2-309, 2-313, 2-315, 2-355, 2-371, 2-384, 2-386, 2-387, 2-405, 2-408, 2-421, 2-464, 2-537, 3-25, 3-27, 3-129, 3-457, 3-460, 3-466, 3-471, 3-504, 3-506–3-509, 3-511, 3-514, 3-516–3-518, 3-523, 3-525, 3-560–3-563, 3-569, 3-570, 3-582–3-587, 3-594, 3-598–3-602, 3-606, 3-609, 3-610, 3-628–3-631, 3-633, 3-636, 3-638–3-645, 3-647–3-656, 3-658–3-663, 3-667
receptor function, 1-399, 1-486, 1-492, 3-25, 3-561

receptor ligands, 2-236
receptor modulators, 2-168
receptor subtypes, 1-237, 1-242, 1-484, 2-96, 2-144, 2-156, 2-238, 2-372, 2-386, 2-387
receptors, 1-xix, 1-xxv, 1-169, 1-171, 1-172, 1-213, 1-215–1-217, 1-223–1-225, 1-236–1-238, 1-241–1-243, 1-245, 1-252, 1-254, 1-255, 1-257, 1-259, 1-260, 1-262–1-265, 1-267–1-269, 1-280, 1-281, 1-284–1-288, 1-292, 1-293, 1-307, 1-312, 1-314, 1-319, 1-323, 1-324, 1-326, 1-343, 1-357, 1-358, 1-369, 1-384, 1-396, 1-399, 1-400, 1-405, 1-422, 1-441, 1-449–1-451, 1-468–1-471, 1-481–1-486, 1-488–1-492, 1-505, 1-506, 1-509, 1-510, 1-528, 1-530, 2-17, 2-46, 2-93, 2-96–2-99, 2-148, 2-150–2-153, 2-156, 2-159, 2-160, 2-171, 2-175–2-177, 2-204, 2-208, 2-235–2-240, 2-245, 2-246, 2-293, 2-312, 2-354, 2-355, 2-368, 2-372, 2-382, 2-386–2-388, 2-397, 2-404, 2-408, 2-420–2-422, 2-425, 2-461, 2-510, 3-69, 3-280, 3-334, 3-453, 3-457, 3-460, 3-461, 3-466, 3-467, 3-476, 3-504–3-509, 3-511, 3-512, 3-514, 3-516, 3-518, 3-521, 3-526, 3-558, 3-567, 3-582, 3-583, 3-587, 3-598–3-602, 3-604–3-606, 3-609, 3-610, 3-626, 3-628–3-631, 3-633, 3-636, 3-638, 3-640, 3-641, 3-643–3-656, 3-658–3-663, 3-665–3-669, 3-764, 3-769, 3-772–3-774, 3-796
    discovery of, 1-169

rectum, 1-123

recurrent depression, *see* major depressive disorder

red bang, *see* cannabis

reducing agent, 2-12, 2-105

reference member state (RMS), 3-51

reflex, 1-139, 1-144, 1-203, 1-213, 1-219, 1-227, 1-229, 2-79, 2-159, 2-220, 2-221, 3-386, 3-607, 3-609

reflex arc, 1-203, 3-598

refractory period, 3-348

Refusal, *see* disulfiram

regeneration, 1-169, 1-199, 1-206, 3-507

regulatory, 1-259, 1-262, 1-281, 1-383, 1-428, 2-225, 2-240, 3-15, 3-42, 3-50, 3-54, 3-55, 3-58, 3-61, 3-64–3-66, 3-68, 3-107, 3-114, 3-137–3-141, 3-161, 3-162, 3-225, 3-232, 3-241, 3-248, 3-252, 3-254, 3-255, 3-476, 3-510, 3-514, 3-516, 3-552, 3-570, 3-610, 3-634, 3-665

Reil, Johann Christian, 1-11, 1-102

Rein, Friedrich Hermann, 3-761

Remak, Robert, 1-188

Remeron, *see* mirtazapine

remission, 1-482–1-484, 1-488, 2-5, 2-59, 2-158, 2-174, 2-176, 2-177, 2-181, 2-185, 2-186, 2-273, 2-406, 3-84, 3-134, 3-310, 3-346, 3-454, 3-462, 3-464, 3-646

spontaneous, 2-4, 2-5, 2-274, 2-275

remoxipride, 1-319, 3-66, 3-128, 3-650, 3-652, 3-659

Renaissance, 1-47, 1-57, 1-59, 1-60, 1-62, 1-64, 1-72, 1-73, 1-183, 2-359, 2-437, 2-446, 2-461, 3-125, 3-435, 3-705, 3-707–3-710, 3-717

renal, 1-294, 1-339, 1-487, 2-187, 2-276, 2-283, 2-511, 3-48, 3-64

renal insufficiency, 2-283, 3-467

repinotan, 2-247

rescinnamine, 2-10

reserpine, 1-154, 1-162, 1-238, 1-240, 1-307, 1-420, 1-459, 1-460, 1-465–1-471, 2-7, 2-10, 2-15, 2-16, **2-23**, 2-23, 2-24, 2-29, 2-32–2-35, 2-37–2-42, 2-44–2-46, 2-80, 2-84, 2-93, 2-94, 2-96, 2-106, 2-107, 2-126, 2-136, 2-142, 2-146, 2-219, 2-454, 3-367, 3-628, 3-761–3-767, 3-769, 3-771, 3-773

adverse effects of, 2-38

non-reserpine neuroleptics, 1-459, 1-468, 1-470, 1-472

reserpine's clinical decline, 2-40

Serpasil, 1-460

resorcine, 1-147

resorcinol, 1-130

respiration, 1-156, 1-157, 1-346, 2-220, 2-354

respiratory center, 1-155

response variable, 1-431, 1-432

reticular formation, 1-220, 1-223, 2-220

retigabine, *see* ezogabine

retina, 1-196, 1-197, 1-199, 1-201

reverse afferentation, 1-215–1-218, 1-220, 1-224, 1-227, 1-228

reverse transcription, 1-278, 3-546

Reynolds, John Russell, 2-461

RGH-188, *see* cariprazine

Rhazes, 1-47, 2-432, 2-511, 3-436, 3-437, 3-439

rhinitis, 2-159

rhodopsin, 1-285, 3-583

Rhovane, *see* zopiclone

RIA, *see* radioimmunoassay (RIA)

ribonucleic acid

RNA, 1-229, 1-278–1-281, 1-296, 3-550, 3-553, 3-564, 3-567–3-

570

Richardson, Benjamin Ward, 2-255
Richelieu, 1-59, 2-439, 2-500
rickets, 1-127, 1-144, 3-429
riluzole, 3-643, 3-644
rimcazole, 3-659
rimonabant, 3-660
    SR-141716, 3-660
Rinkel, Max, 2-534
risperidone, 1-314, 1-358, 1-361, 1-364,
       2-98, 2-192, 2-193, 2-197,
       2-366, 3-133, 3-134, 3-218,
       3-252, 3-308, 3-474, 3-650,
       3-653, 3-658, 3-661
    9-OH-risperidone, 3-649
Ritalin, *see* methylphenidate
ritanserin, 3-652
rivastigmine, 2-383–2-385
Rivea corymbosa, *see* ololiuqui
RNA, *see* ribonucleic acid
RNA editing, 1-286
RNA polymerase, 3-570
RNA processing, 3-568
Ro 15-1788, *see* flumazenil
RO 5-0690, *see* chlordiazepoxide
Robert H. Collyer, 2-443
Robert-Fluery, Tony, *1-5*
Robertis, Eduardo De, 1-206
Robins, Eli, 1-26, 3-324
Robinson, Leslie, 3-9
Robinson, Robert, 2-31
Rocket Fuel, *see* phencyclidine
rod, 1-416, 1-513
Rohypnol, *see* flunitrazepam
rolipram, 3-635, 3-637
Romanov, Miguel, 2-500
Roosevelt, Theodore, 3-192
Roquet, Salvador, 2-537
Rossignol, P., 2-82
Rousseau, Jean-Jacques, 3-706
RP-27267, *see* zopiclone
RP-62204, *see* fananserin
Rubiaceae, 2-456

Rubio, Eduardo Sánchez, 1-129
Rubio, Gabriel, 1-xxviii
Rubio, Pedro M., 3-720
Runge, Ferdinand, 1-346, 2-531
rupture, 1-18
Rush, Benjamin, 2-305, 2-333, 3-381
Russian sthenosina Orel, 1-145
Rutherford, Daniel, 2-440

S

Séglas, Jules, 1-18
Sérieux, Paul, 1-12
S-15535, *see* alnespirone
sabcomeline, 3-654
    SB 202026, 3-654
Sabuco, Miguel, 1-50
Safeguard, *see* diclofenac
safety, 1-385, 1-415, 1-418, 1-421–1-424,
       1-429, 1-447, 2-7, 2-40, 2-44,
       2-105, 2-111, 2-112, 2-157,
       2-158, 2-171, 2-211, 2-220,
       2-233, 2-256, 2-293, 2-295,
       2-384, 2-510, 2-547, 2-556,
       3-15, 3-48–3-50, 3-53, 3-55,
       3-56, 3-58, 3-61, 3-64, 3-65,
       3-67, 3-80, 3-107, 3-121,
       3-127, 3-130, 3-139–3-142,
       3-156, 3-161, 3-165, 3-166,
       3-218, 3-234, 3-246, 3-255,
       3-277, 3-306, 3-307, 3-311,
       3-345, 3-352, 3-354, 3-389,
       3-463, 3-471, 3-626, 3-628,
       3-641, 3-642, 3-647, 3-660,
       3-662, 3-765
Saint Anthony, 2-461
Sakel, Manfred J., 3-344
Sakel, Manfred Joshua, 2-276
salicin, 1-130
Salvarsan, *see* arsphenamine
Salvia, 2-466, 2-538
    Shepherd's Leaf, 2-538
Salvia divinorum, *see* Salvia
Salzmann, M.M., 2-132

Sandison, Ronald A., 2-536

sandoptal, 1-160

Sapindaceae, 2-456

Saponaria, 1-130

sarcosine, 3-657

    N-methylglycine, 3-508

saredutant, 3-647

Saroten, *see* amitriptyline

Saulle, Henri Legrand du, 1-14

SB 202026, *see* sabcomeline

Schedule I, 2-481, 3-22

Schedule II, 3-55, 3-68

Schedule III, 3-24, 3-55

Schedule IV, 3-55

Schild, H.O., 1-171

Schildkraut, Joseph, 2-137

Schindler, W., 2-126

schizophrenia, 1-ix, 1-xv, 1-11, 1-13,
    1-18, 1-19, 1-23, 1-167, 1-238,
    1-245, 1-263, 1-284, 1-291–
    1-293, 1-296, 1-319, 1-357,
    1-358, 1-400, 1-401, 1-403–
    1-406, 1-418, 1-421, 1-446,
    1-448, 1-459, 1-460, 1-462,
    1-463, 1-465, 1-466, 1-468,
    1-470–1-472, 1-480, 1-493,
    1-527, 2-4, 2-5, 2-8, 2-10,
    2-17, 2-26, 2-33, 2-35, 2-38,
    2-44–2-46, 2-65, 2-67, 2-85,
    2-93–2-100, 2-136, 2-193,
    2-229, 2-230, 2-232, 2-335,
    2-336, 2-339, 2-340, 2-342,
    2-343, 2-355, 2-399, 2-401,
    2-402, 2-404, 2-405, 2-407,
    2-408, 2-448, 2-454, 2-514,
    2-524, 2-525, 2-532, 2-533,
    3-5, 3-10, 3-11, 3-22–3-24,
    3-27, 3-37, 3-52, 3-61, 3-70,
    3-83, 3-84, 3-89, 3-90, 3-113,
    3-132–3-135, 3-174, 3-176,
    3-228, 3-233, 3-235, 3-247,
    3-278, 3-280, 3-282, 3-293,
    3-296, 3-297, 3-306, 3-308,
    3-310, 3-316, 3-323, 3-328,
    3-330, 3-333–3-335, 3-344,
    3-347, 3-385, 3-417, 3-495,
    3-504–3-509, 3-511, 3-516,
    3-518, 3-520–3-523, 3-527,
    3-543, 3-545, 3-551, 3-552,
    3-563, 3-570, 3-582, 3-587,
    3-611, 3-648–3-656, 3-658–
    3-661, 3-731, 3-745, 3-748,
    3-749, 3-766, 3-773–3-775,
    3-790, 3-793

    "coffee groups", 2-533

    amphetamine model, 1-405

    disorganized, 2-80

    model, 3-23, 3-24, 3-518

schizophrenics, 1-162, 1-314, 2-17,
    2-245, 2-274, 2-275, 2-406,
    2-407, 3-563, 3-655, 3-661

schizotypal personality disorder, 3-333

Schlittler, Emil, 2-30, 2-454

Schmidt, Paul, 2-135

Schmiedeberg, Oswald, 1-110, 1-111, 1-
    234, 1-235, 3-757

Schneider, 1-xv, 1-190, 3-99, 3-100, 3-
    333, 3-362, 3-747, 3-750, 3-766

Schneider, Carl, 3-92, 3-97, 3-99, 3-100

Schneider, Jean, 2-60

Schou, Mogens, 1-380, 2-7, 2-168,
    2-185, 3-14

Schultes, Richard Evans, 2-432, 3-795

Schultze, E., 1-135, 1-190

Schwann, Theodor, 1-187

SCL, *see* Symptom Checklist (SCL)

scleroderma, 2-402

scopolamine, 1-146, 1-155, 1-158,
    2-4, 2-58, 2-266, 2-274, 2-
    306, 2-307, 2-328, 2-361,
    2-362, 2-386, 2-434, 2-445,
    2-447–2-449, 3-235, 3-499,
    3-762

    hyoscine, 1-146, 1-147, 1-151, 2-4,
    2-266, 2-306, 2-328, 2-359, 2-
    361, 2-362

scopolamine bromhydrate, 1-160
scopolamine bromhydrate, *see* scopolamine
scotoma, 1-88
Scott, Walter, 2-439, 3-492
scrofula, 1-137, 1-144
scurvy, 1-416
seasonal affective disorder, 1-492, 3-520
secobarbital, 1-506, 2-272, 2-279, 2-281,
2-285
Seconal, 1-160, 1-506, 2-272
Seconal, *see* secobarbital
Second International Opium Convention, *see* opium
second messenger, 1-171, 1-245, 1-250,
1-254, 1-257, 1-269, 1-447,
2-248, 3-512, 3-514, 3-518,
3-598, 3-600, 3-630, 3-631
second messenger systems, 1-268
secretin, 3-661
sedative, 1-xxv, 1-xxvii, 1-68, 1-94,
1-104, 1-108, 1-109, 1-119,
1-123, 1-128, 1-134, 1-136,
1-143, 1-147, 1-149, 1-151–
1-153, 1-155, 1-158–1-160,
1-168, 1-229, 1-307, 1-308,
1-319, 1-323, 1-324, 1-326,
1-331, 1-336, 1-337, 1-339,
1-341, 1-352, 1-395, 1-420,
1-460, 1-506, 1-509, 2-4, 2-8,
2-9, 2-13, 2-16, 2-27–2-31,
2-33, 2-44, 2-56, 2-58, 2-60,
2-65, 2-79, 2-80, 2-86, 2-94,
2-111, 2-126, 2-132, 2-137,
2-191, 2-194, 2-203, 2-220,
2-229–2-231, 2-233, 2-236,
2-239, 2-248, 2-256, 2-258,
2-265–2-267, 2-269, 2-270,
2-272, 2-278, 2-283, 2-286,
2-294–2-296, 2-298, 2-299,
2-306, 2-311, 2-326, 2-328,
2-329, 2-334, 2-359–2-364,
2-438, 2-454, 2-455, 2-495,
2-496, 2-506, 2-512, 2-513,
2-515, 2-524, 2-555–2-561,
3-6, 3-8, 3-9, 3-25, 3-67, 3-130,
3-180, 3-189, 3-210, 3-215,
3-235, 3-277, 3-361, 3-365,
3-368, 3-452, 3-457, 3-459,
3-466, 3-474, 3-475, 3-649,
3-662, 3-663, 3-665, 3-666,
3-685, 3-765
seemetamizole, 3-299, 3-771
seizures, 1-144, 1-328–1-331, 1-333–
1-335, 1-379, 1-506, 1-512–
1-514, 2-113, 2-208, 2-210,
2-239, 2-260, 2-265, 2-277,
2-278, 2-283, 2-285, 2-329,
2-336–2-338, 2-350, 2-559,
3-25, 3-54, 3-84, 3-211, 3-344,
3-415, 3-604, 3-740
selective serotonin reuptake inhibitor
(SSRI), 1-295, 1-341, 1-343,
1-352, 1-356, 1-357, 1-448,
1-450, 1-484, 1-485, 1-488,
1-490, 1-491, 2-110, 2-125,
2-137, 2-138, 2-141, 2-150,
2-152–2-156, 2-159, 2-160,
2-171–2-177, 2-197, 2-240,
2-313, 2-347, 2-367, 2-368,
3-42, 3-83, 3-131, 3-132,
3-227, 3-244–3-246, 3-278,
3-313–3-316, 3-332, 3-333,
3-354, 3-453–3-457, 3-460,
3-462, 3-464, 3-468, 3-471,
3-517, 3-626, 3-628, 3-630,
3-631, 3-634, 3-636, 3-638,
3-642, 3-644, 3-664, 3-666
selegiline, 1-340, 2-112, 2-353
deprenyl, 1-340, 2-112, 2-353
L-deprenyl, 2-112
Selfotel (CGS-19755), 3-656
Selye, Hans, 2-56, 2-397
semagacestat, 2-390
semen, 2-435, 2-508
Semmelweis, Ignaz, 2-431

Sen, Gananath, 2-28, 2-453

Senecio, 1-146

seproxetine

    norfluoxetine, 2-147, 2-148, 2-150

septum, 1-223

sequential design, 1-434

Serax, *see* oxazepam

serendipity, 1-xii, 1-xix, 1-xxv, 1-179, 1-356, 2-204, 2-276, 3-359–3-361, 3-363, 3-364, 3-367–3-369

Seresta, *see* oxazepam

serial analysis of gene expression (SAGE), 2-466, 3-546

Sernyl, *see* phencyclidine

Sernylan, *see* phencyclidine

serotonin, 1-162, 1-205, 1-238, 1-240, 1-242, 1-249, 1-254, 1-280, 1-286, 1-304, 1-314, 1-319, 1-321, 1-336, 1-339–1-341, 1-343, 1-356, 1-357, 1-399, 1-421, 1-423, 1-424, 1-450, 1-459, 1-460, 1-462, 1-463, 1-465, 1-466, 1-468, 1-471, 1-480, 2-14, 2-15, 2-44, 2-46, 2-93, 2-95, 2-96, 2-99, 2-100, 2-106, 2-113, 2-114, 2-137, 2-141, 2-156, 2-167, 2-247, 2-248, 2-313, 2-350, 2-355, 2-357, 2-537, 3-65, 3-69, 3-131, 3-144, 3-218, 3-277, 3-312, 3-418, 3-451, 3-453–3-455, 3-459, 3-460, 3-467, 3-471, 3-505, 3-506, 3-510, 3-511, 3-514, 3-521, 3-523, 3-525, 3-595, 3-598, 3-610, 3-612, 3-625, 3-626, 3-628, 3-630, 3-634, 3-652, 3-654, 3-665, 3-762, 3-763, 3-765, 3-771

    5-HT, 1-286, 1-295, 1-304, 1-356, 1-357, 1-367–1-369, 1-460, 1-463, 1-480–1-487, 1-489, 1-493, 1-495, 1-514, 2-15,

2-16, 2-106, 2-107, 2-111, 2-142, 2-144, 2-146–2-148, 2-150–2-154, 2-157, 2-158, 2-160, 2-161, 2-167, 2-168, 2-171, 2-173–2-176, 2-245, 2-313, 2-368, 2-370, 3-506, 3-600, 3-649, 3-665, 3-774

5-HT$_{1A}$, 1-257, 1-286, 1-312, 1-314, 1-326, 1-352, 1-369, 1-395, 1-450, 1-482–1-487, 1-514, 2-98, 2-152–2-154, 2-246, 2-247, 2-368, 2-370, 3-506, 3-630, 3-649, 3-654, 3-665

5-HT$_{1B}$, 1-483

5-HT$_{1D}$, 1-314, 1-483

5-HT$_1$, 1-286, 1-357, 1-483, 1-495, 2-156, 3-772

5-HT$_{2A}$, 1-294, 1-295, 1-312, 1-314, 1-357, 1-369, 1-450, 1-483, 2-93, 2-96, 2-98, 2-99, 3-506, 3-511, 3-652, 3-653

5-HT$_{2B}$, 3-653

5-HT$_{2C}$, 1-294, 1-295, 1-312, 1-483, 2-150, 2-152, 2-245, 3-506, 3-648, 3-653

5-HT$_2$, 1-259, 1-357, 1-358, 1-395, 1-483, 1-493, 2-96–2-98, 2-156, 2-175, 2-355, 3-69, 3-506, 3-611, 3-626, 3-630, 3-652, 3-653, 3-773

5-HT$_3$, 1-268, 1-286, 1-312, 1-319, 1-357, 1-395, 2-156, 2-175, 2-176, 2-204, 3-653, 3-665, 3-666

5-HT$_4$, 1-369

5-HT$_6$, 1-294, 1-312, 3-653

5-HT$_7$, 1-286, 1-312, 1-483, 3-654

serotonin syndrome, 2-114

serotonin-norepinephrine reuptake inhibitor (SNRI), 1-343, 2-168, 2-171, 2-174, 2-176, 3-457, 3-517, 3-626

Serpasil, *see* reserpine

serpent, 3-395, 3-396, 3-407

serpentine, 2-10, 2-27, 2-30, 2-46

serpentinine, 2-30

Sertürner, 2-3, 2-416, 2-442, 2-443, 2-475

Sertürner, Friedrich Wilhelm, 1-110, 1-303, 2-266, 2-416, 2-442, 2-453

Sertürner, W.A., 2-509

sertindole, 2-98, **3-68**, 3-68, 3-299, 3-310

sertraline, 1-343, 1-352, 1-356, 1-361, 2-141, 2-157, 2-158, 2-174–2-176, 2-310, 2-313, 3-246, 3-453, 3-468, 3-471, 3-642, 3-644, 3-645

    Zoloft, 2-310

serum, 1-93, 1-94, 1-140, 1-159, 1-160, 1-359, 1-375–1-380, 1-384, 1-385, 1-409, 1-460, 2-185, 2-233, 2-279, 2-307, 2-497, 3-311, 3-508, 3-639, 3-646, 3-775

sexual dysfunction, 1-357, 2-171, 2-524, 3-246

Shakespeare, William, 2-438, 3-494

Shaw, Thomas Claye, 2-342

Sheehan Disability Scale, 3-315

Shen Nung, 2-482

Shepherd's Leaf, *see* Salvia

Shepherd, M., 2-35

Sherrington, Charles, 1-219

Sherrington, Charles Scott, 1-169, 1-203

shock, 1-21, 1-113, 1-267, 1-420, 2-55, 2-56, 2-60, 2-61, 2-71, 2-81, 2-222, 2-225, 2-276, 2-279, 2-325, 2-331, 2-332, 2-405, 3-6, 3-343, 3-344, 3-361, 3-362, 3-368, 3-475, 3-561

shock therapy, 1-19, 2-37, 2-65, 2-66, 2-125, 2-338, 3-327

    cardiazol, 2-272

    ducking, 2-332

    insulin, 2-272

Shore, Parkhurst A., 2-44

Shorter, Edward, 1-28, 2-266

sibutramine, 1-343, 2-350, 3-471

Siddiqui, Rafat Hussain, 2-30

Siddiqui, Salimuz Zaman, 2-30

Sierra, Miguel Rojo, 3-716

Sieveking, Edward Henry, 2-259

sigma receptor, 3-658, 3-659

sigma receptors, 2-421, 3-658

signal transduction, 1-171, 1-250, 1-257, 1-264, 1-269, 1-280, 1-284, 3-509, 3-510, 3-512, 3-514, 3-518, 3-521, 3-525–3-527, 3-560, 3-564, 3-585, 3-631, 3-633, 3-638

silver albuminate, 1-146

Similie, E.R., 2-443

Simon, 1-37, 1-242, 3-175

Simpson, James Young, 1-305, 2-256, 2-444

Sinequan, *see* doxepin

single nucleotide polymorphism (SNP), 1-282, 1-289–1-291, 1-293, 1-384, 3-507, 3-512, 3-517, 3-520, 3-544, 3-545, 3-550, 3-567, 3-582

single-photon emission computed tomography (SPECT), 1-352, 1-368, 1-369, 1-448–1-450, 1-492, 3-349, 3-401, 3-505

skeletal muscle, 1-234, 1-346, 2-561, 3-5

skeletal muscle paralysis, 3-349

skeletal muscle relaxation, 2-220, 2-221

Slater, Eliot, 2-276

sleep apnea, 3-461

    obstructive, 2-296

sleep disorders, 1-324, 2-40, 2-265, 2-266, 2-295, 2-297, 3-65, 3-247

small intestine, 2-283, 3-495

smooth muscle, 1-260, 1-346, 1-463

snakeroot, *see* Rauwofia serpentina

Snell, 1-11

Snow, John, 2-444

Snyder, S.H., 1-171

social adaptation, 3-306, 3-312, 3-313, 3-315, 3-316

social adjustment, 3-306, 3-468

Socrates, 3-379

sodium, 1-129, 1-138, 1-140, 1-141, 1-147, 1-148, 1-151, 1-152, 1-159, 1-160, 1-329, 1-334, 1-335, 1-380, 2-63, 2-191–2-193, 2-204, 2-210, 2-257, 2-278, 2-281, 2-283, 2-307, 2-313, 2-364, 2-555, 3-278, 3-460, 3-496, 3-598, 3-602

sodium amytal, 1-xxv, 1-160, 2-279

sodium barbital, *see* barbital

sodium benzoate, 1-160, 2-532

sodium bromide, 1-151, 2-260, 2-363

sodium cacodylate, 1-152

sodium glycerophosphate, 1-140, 1-144

sodium hypobromite, 1-148

sodium pentothal, *see* thiopental

sodium persulfate, 1-152

sodium phosphate, 1-140, 1-144

sodium salicylate, 1-130, 1-151

sodium thiopental, *see* thiopental

Solanaceae, *see* nightshade (Solanaceae)

Solanaceaes, 1-129, 2-445, 2-447, 2-498

solanezumab, 2-391

Solomon, George F., 2-398

Soma, *see* carisoprodol

somatic, 1-19, 1-21, 1-40, 1-41, 1-60, 1-102, 1-105, 1-106, 1-112, 1-216, 2-176, 2-340, 2-364, 2-368, 2-369, 2-551, 3-226, 3-229, 3-282, 3-328, 3-333, 3-447, 3-455–3-457, 3-459, 3-463, 3-467, 3-568, 3-661, 3-705, 3-706, 3-711, 3-736

somatization, 3-315

somatostatin, 3-601, 3-610, 3-647

Somnifen, 1-158, **2-4**, 2-272–2-275, 2-278

Sonal, 1-149

soporific, 1-139, 1-147, 1-460, 1-528, 2-3, 2-436–2-438, 2-449, 2-455, 2-506, 3-439

Spaltung, 1-18

sparteine, 1-130, 1-160, 2-307

spasm, 1-73, 3-346

spasms, 1-73, 1-127, 1-131, 1-322, 2-448, 2-519, 3-476

Spath, E., 2-534

special K, *see* ketamine

Specific benzodiazepine receptors were discovered in the brain in 1977, 1-509

SPECT, *see* single-photon emission computed tomography (SPECT)

spermatorrhea, 1-136

spinal cord, 1-124, 1-127, 1-128, 1-157, 1-168, 1-184, 1-191, 1-196, 1-199, 1-213, 1-481, 1-488, 1-491, 2-221, 2-234, 3-135, 3-598, 3-601, 3-604, 3-645

spinal fractures, 3-349

Spitzer, Robert L., 1-26, 3-324

Spivey, 2-519

spleen, 2-511, 3-730, 3-732

Sprenger, Dominicans Jacob, 2-435

SR-141716, *see* rimonabant

St. John's wort (Hypericum perfora-tum), 1-351, 1-352, 1-358, 1-359, **1-364**, 1-364–1-366, 1-370, 2-458, 3-584

Störck, Anton, 1-69

Staff, *see* etoperidone

Stanford Jr., Leland, 3-169

Stanton, Joseph R., 2-29

starvation, 3-95

statistical analysis, 1-427, 1-429–1-431

status epilepticus, 1-334, 2-286

Steck, Hans, 2-38

Steenhauer, J., 2-29

Sterculiaceae, 2-456

Sternbach, Leo, 1-322, 1-506, 2-365, 3-504, 3-792
Sternbach, Leo H., 2-231
steroid, 1-268, 3-584, 3-605
Stevens-Johnson syndrome, 2-196, 2-206
Stevenson, 2-528
stimulant, 1-112, 1-118, 1-146, 1-150, 1-154, 1-160, 1-162, 1-168, 1-205, 1-345, 1-347, 1-349, 1-350, 1-395, 1-403, 1-459, 1-469, 1-470, 1-472, 1-479, 1-528, 1-530, 2-111, 2-220, 2-286, 2-326, 2-330, 2-348–2-351, 2-354, 2-355, 2-448, 2-458, 2-479, 2-480, 2-495, 2-496, 2-513, 2-523, 2-524, 2-527, 2-528, 2-535, 2-545, 3-54, 3-69, 3-198, 3-209, 3-210, 3-213–3-215, 3-226, 3-244, 3-245, 3-247, 3-374, 3-498, 3-599, 3-660, 3-773, 3-796
stimulation, 1-186, 1-205, 1-222, 1-223, 1-225–1-228, 1-234, 1-235, 1-257, 1-259, 1-260, 1-267, 1-283, 1-403, 1-407–1-409, 1-470, 1-483, 1-485, 1-495, 1-528, 1-530, 2-152, 2-175, 2-329, 2-347–2-349, 2-357, 2-386, 2-388, 2-422, 3-88, 3-346, 3-351, 3-353, 3-355, 3-364, 3-384, 3-459, 3-474, 3-516, 3-610, 3-645, 3-659, 3-662, 3-667, 3-764, 3-775, 3-796
Stoll, 2-544–2-547
Stoll, Arthur, 2-461, 2-544, 2-548
Stoll, Werner A, 2-535, 2-548
stomach, 1-41, 1-44, 1-48, 1-93, 1-121, 1-123, 1-124, 1-128, 1-132, 1-135, 1-137, 1-140, 1-150, 1-151, 1-528, 2-176, 2-283, 2-448, 2-513, 3-495, 3-732

Stopetyl, *see* disulfiram
stratified, 1-433
stress disorders
    post-traumatic, 2-549
stroke, 2-387, 3-740
strontium bromide, 1-132, 1-146
Strophanthus, 1-130
Strube, Georg, 2-510
strychnine, 1-108, 1-110, 1-119, 1-131, 1-138, 1-140, 1-141, 1-143, 1-144, 1-154, 1-157, 1-159, 1-377, 1-511, 1-512, 2-191, 2-305–2-307, 3-344, 3-604, 3-610
stuttering, 3-448
Suavitil, *see* benactyzine
subarachnoid space, 1-442
Suboxone, *see* buprenorphine
substance abuse, 3-83, 3-138, 3-174, 3-207, 3-226, 3-232, 3-325, 3-417, 3-420, 3-447, 3-524, 3-685
substrate, 1-161, 1-252, 1-259, 1-340, 1-527, 1-530, 2-14, 2-15, 2-111, 2-222, 2-458, 3-333, 3-548, 3-560, 3-610
Subutex, *see* buprenorphine
succinyl norcocaine, 2-314
    cocaine vaccine, 2-314
succinylcholine, 2-308, 2-338, 3-349
sucralfate, 3-465
suicide, 1-6, 1-335, 1-340, 1-486, 1-490, 1-493, 2-40, 2-132, 2-220, 2-282, 2-415, 2-443, 2-462, 2-537, 2-549, 2-558, 3-42, 3-64, 3-77, 3-81, 3-83, 3-100, 3-114, 3-121, 3-132, 3-199, 3-218, 3-245, 3-246, 3-250, 3-299, 3-310, 3-314, 3-316, 3-336, 3-352, 3-388, 3-492, 3-499, 3-511, 3-518, 3-520, 3-522, 3-523, 3-645
sulfate, 1-152, 2-127

sulfomethanes, 1-160

sulfonal, 1-119, 1-134, 1-135, 1-137, 1-139, 1-140, 1-146, 1-149, 1-151, 1-156, 1-158, 1-352, 2-267, 2-269, 2-272

sulpiride, 1-319, 1-361, 1-492

Super Acid, *see* ketamine

Super C, *see* ketamine

Super Weed, *see* phencyclidine

superficial, 1-18, 1-122, 3-25, 3-326, 3-498, 3-631

suppression, 1-44, 1-45, 1-73, 1-222, 1-267, 1-397, 1-508, 2-156, 2-256, 2-333, 2-425, 2-431, 2-432, 2-438, 2-442, 3-331, 3-522, 3-523, 3-773, 3-775

    genetic, 1-405

surgery

    brain, 1-19

    frontal lobectomy, 2-342

Surmontil, *see* trimipramine

Swain, Gladys, 1-3, 1-95

Sydenham, Thomas, 1-67, 1-159, 2-362, 2-405, 2-414, 2-439, 2-452, 2-472, 2-508, 2-511, 3-327, 3-374

Symmetrel, *see* amantadine

sympathetic, 1-107, 1-108, 1-121, 1-199, 1-234, 1-235, 1-240, 1-241, 1-243, 1-469, 1-488, 2-14, 2-44, 2-398, 2-399, 3-15, 3-381, 3-596, 3-757, 3-764

sympathin, 2-14

sympathomimetic amine, 2-110, 3-765

Symptom Checklist (SCL), 3-303, 3-305–3-307, 3-315

synapse, 1-202–1-204, 1-206, 1-208, 1-219, 1-307, 1-341, 2-14, 2-15, 3-593

synapsin II, 1-295

synaptic transmission, 1-172, 1-205, 1-233, 1-253, 1-254, 1-262, 1-264, 2-387, 3-628, 3-630, 3-658

synergistic, 1-253, 1-293, 2-112, 3-401, 3-403, 3-513, 3-797

syphilis, 1-62, 1-132, 1-137, 1-141, 2-339, 2-407, 3-89, 3-280, 3-720

Syrup of the infant Jesus, 1-142

systemic, 1-241, 1-446, 2-152, 2-325, 3-225, 3-232, 3-562

Szasz, Thomas S., 1-22, 3-231, 3-283

T

T4, *see* thyroxine

Tabern, Donalee L., 2-272

Tabernanthe iboga, *see* iboga

tachycardia, 2-159, 2-275, 3-299

tacrine, 2-383

tactile, 1-38, 1-225, 2-530

tallina, 1-130

tamoxifen , 1-331

tandem affinity purification, 3-558

tandospirone, 2-246

Tanzi, Eugenio, 3-714

TAP, 3-558

Tardieu, Y., 2-10, 2-34

tarenflurbil, 2-390

target organ, 3-281

TCP, *see* tenocyclidine

tea, 1-335, 1-346, 1-460, 2-354, 2-456–2-458, 2-496, 2-515, 2-523, 2-532, 3-190

Tegretol, *see* carbamazepine

telangiectasia, 3-547

telemedicine, 3-620

temazepam, 2-295, 3-217

Temposil, *see* disulfiram

tendon, 3-607

tenocyclidine, 3-22

    TCP, 3-22, 3-26, 3-615, 3-616

Tenuf, 2-432

teonanácatl, *see* peyote

Terenius, Lars, 1-242

testosterone, 3-647

tetanus, 1-121, 1-133, 1-141, 1-157, 2-286, 2-447, 2-448, 2-510
tetany, 1-318
tetrabamate, 3-68
   Atrium, 3-774
tetrahydrocannabinol (THC), 2-447, 2-449, 2-484, 2-515, 2-520, 2-522, 3-660
   delta-9-THC, 2-520, 2-521
   dronabinol, 2-521, 3-660
   Marinol, 2-521
tetrahydrocannabinol (THC) receptors, 2-461
tetrahydroharmine (THH), 2-445
tetrahydroisoquinolic alkaloids, 2-449
tetronal, 1-135, 1-136, 1-139, 1-146, 1-149
thalamus, 1-220, 2-151, 2-222, 3-598
thalidomide, 1-331, 1-422, 2-81, 2-133, 3-15, 3-49, 3-58, 3-64
The Belmont Report, 3-105, 3-154
Theaceae, 2-456
thebaine, 1-131, 2-416, 3-344, 3-491
Theobald, W., 2-136
Theobroma cacao, see cacao (Theobroma cacao)
theobromine, 1-153, 1-346, 2-531
Theodoric of Cervia, 2-436
theophylline, 1-346, 2-286, 2-531
   Aminophylline, 1-346
theory of exclusion, 3-347
theory of seduction, 1-16
therapeutic adherence, 3-179
therapeutic drug monitoring, 1-361, 1-375, 1-378, 1-379, 1-382, 1-384
thiamine deficiency, 2-5
Thiebaux, M., 2-38
Thiele, J., 2-126
thiohydantoin, 1-332
thionembutal, see thiopental
thiopental, 2-272, 2-279, 2-283, 2-286, 3-350
   Pentothal, 2-63, 2-64, 2-272, 2-279

sodium pentothal, 2-279, 3-496
sodium pentothal narcosis, 2-307
sodium thiopental, 2-279, 2-281, 2-284
thionembutal, 2-278
thiophene, 1-324, 1-331
thioridazine, 1-311, 1-360, 2-17, 2-98, 3-69, 3-70, 3-299
thiothixene, 2-86
Thorazine, see chlorpromazine (CPZ)
thrombocytopenia, 3-64
thrombosis, 2-40
Thuillier, Jean, 2-65, 3-359, 3-363, 3-790
thuja, 1-130
Thutmose IV, 3-435
thymacetine, 1-135, 1-146, 1-151
thyroxine, 3-763
   T4, 3-94
tiagabine, 2-208, 2-209, 3-664
tianeptine, 3-628
tics, 1-132, 1-141, 3-448, 3-476
time-of-flight mass spectrometer, 3-556
Tinbergen, Nikolaas, 1-226, 3-413
tincture of opium, see laudanum
tinea, 1-123
tissue, 1-168, 1-169, 1-172, 1-186, 1-187, 1-191, 1-219, 1-254, 1-259, 1-279, 1-442, 1-447, 1-469, 1-472, 2-60, 2-61, 2-111, 2-150, 2-267, 2-283, 2-284, 2-398, 2-402, 3-9, 3-526, 3-527, 3-547, 3-551–3-554, 3-556, 3-563, 3-568, 3-610
Tito, Arnaudi, 3-498
TMS, see Transcranial Magnetic Stimulation (TMS)
TNF, see tumor necrosis factor (TNF)
tobacco, 1-66, 1-119, 1-122, 1-123, 1-130, 1-146, 1-160, 2-458, 2-473, 2-476, 2-489, 2-498–2-501, 2-508, 2-524, 2-525, 3-22, 3-24, 3-41, 3-188, 3-464, 3-655
snuff, 3-797

Tofranil, *see* imipramine

tolerability, 2-132, 2-133, 2-138, 2-169–2-171, 2-206, 3-308, 3-453, 3-472, 3-473, 3-628, 3-644, 3-647, 3-649, 3-652

tolerance, 1-131, 1-343, 1-352, 1-406, 1-407, 1-422, 1-424, 1-495, 2-37, 2-79, 2-177, 2-220, 2-222, 2-240, 2-246, 2-277, 2-285, 2-295, 2-298, 2-299, 2-354, 2-366, 2-425, 2-453, 2-473, 2-514, 2-559, 2-561, 3-22, 3-68, 3-69, 3-217, 3-300, 3-348, 3-462, 3-474, 3-496, 3-498, 3-771

toloxatone, 1-341, 1-357

Tolvin, *see* mianserin

tongue, 2-63, 2-175, 3-730

tonic, 1-72, 1-73, 1-104, 1-112, 1-123, 1-127, 1-143, 1-145, 1-149, 1-150, 1-152, 1-153, 1-159, 1-328, 1-331, 1-367, 2-327, 2-329, 2-458, 2-494, 2-496, 2-528, 3-198, 3-346

tooth, 1-134, 2-440, 2-442, 2-443, 2-445, 3-359, 3-360

toothache, 2-499, 2-517, 2-527, 3-439

topiramate, 1-335, 1-379, 1-531, 2-208, 2-210, 2-313, 2-367

Torsades de Pointes, 3-68, 3-69

Tourette syndrome, 2-367

Tourette, Georges Gilles de la, 1-15

toxin, 1-111, 2-183, 2-497, 2-513

tract, 1-108, 1-224, 1-225, 1-227, 2-330, 3-600, 3-601

tramadol, 1-343, 3-454

tranquilizer, 1-xxv, 1-93, 1-118, 1-124, 1-137, 1-139, 1-142, 1-146, 1-148, 1-149, 1-154–1-156, 1-162, 1-309, 1-316, 1-319, 1-322, 1-323, 1-326, 1-420, 1-460, 2-27, 2-29, 2-32, 2-59, 2-61, 2-111, 2-222, 2-223, 2-225, 2-231, 2-311, 2-365, 2-454, 2-509, 2-555, 3-9, 3-189, 3-305, 3-315, 3-381, 3-594, 3-763

Transcranial Magnetic Stimulation (TMS), 3-353, 3-355

transcription, 1-252, 1-257, 1-265, 1-267, 1-268, 2-408, 3-513, 3-518, 3-525–3-527, 3-546, 3-552, 3-553, 3-558, 3-564–3-566, 3-568–3-570, 3-610, 3-631, 3-633–3-635, 3-774

    genetic, 3-634

transcriptome, 3-546, 3-553, 3-583

transcriptomics, 1-291, 3-546

transformation, 1-23, 1-24, 1-107, 1-154, 1-317, 1-378, 2-76, 2-490, 3-600

transgenic animals, 1-406, 2-390

translocation, 1-293, 3-517

Tranxene, *see* clorazepate

tranylcypromine, 1-341, 1-360, 2-12, 2-107–2-110, 2-113, 2-114, 2-353, 3-634, 3-642

trauma, 1-15, 2-56, 2-387, 2-389, 3-228, 3-238, 3-245, 3-413, 3-604

traxoprodil
    CP-101,606, 3-644

trazodone, 2-171, 3-453, 3-626, 3-644

treatment adherence, 3-174

Treaty of Nanking, *see* Opium Wars

tremor, 1-467, 2-193

trephining, 2-341, 3-375

trequinsin, 3-635, 3-638

triazolam, 2-233, 2-240, 2-295, 2-297, 2-299, **3-64**, 3-64, 3-65, 3-217
    Halcion, 2-233, 2-240, 3-64

triazolobenzodiazepine, 3-217

trichloroacetic acid, 2-257

trichloromethyl dithiochloride, 2-257

trichotillomania, 2-160

tricyclic antidepressant (TCA), 1-ix, 1-22, 1-321, 1-335, 1-336,

1-339, 1-341, 1-343, 1-356, 1-357, 1-375, 1-378, 1-382, 1-383, 1-421, 1-423, 1-479, 1-490, 1-491, 2-93, 2-96, 2-111–2-113, 2-125, 2-129, 2-131–2-133, 2-135–2-138, 2-142, 2-144, 2-146, 2-147, 2-150, 2-152, 2-156, 2-159, 2-167, 2-168, 2-170–2-174, 2-176, 2-177, 2-197, 2-310, 2-367, 3-3, 3-11, 3-26, 3-64, 3-121, 3-131, 3-132, 3-218, 3-277, 3-278, 3-312–3-316, 3-354, 3-448, 3-450–3-457, 3-459–3-464, 3-466, 3-504, 3-510, 3-517, 3-610, 3-612, 3-625, 3-626, 3-628, 3-631, 3-634, 3-640, 3-642, 3-644, 3-765, 3-768, 3-770

trihexyphenidyl, 3-762

Trileptal, *see* oxcarbazepine

Trilteptal, *see* oxcarbazepine

trimethadione, 1-333, 2-278

trimethylamine, 1-130

trimipramine, 1-336, 1-360, 2-132, 2-135, 2-137, 3-464, 3-465

Surmontil, 2-132

trinitrine, *see* nitroglycerin

trional, 1-135, 1-136, 1-139, 1-141, 1-146, 1-149, 1-151, 1-156–1-158, 2-306

triphenine, 1-146

tropomyosin, 3-636

trunk, 3-294

trypsin, 3-556

tryptophan (L-trypophan), 1-481–1-484, 1-493, 2-6, 2-16, 2-106, 2-144, 2-152, 2-156, 3-66, 3-467, 3-511, 3-523, 3-525, 3-646

tuberculosis, 1-131, 1-340, 1-352, 1-419, 2-106, 2-275, 2-494, 2-510, 2-528, 3-278, 3-368

pulmonary, 1-122, 1-144, 1-417

tubocurarine

d-tubocurarine, 2-221

Tucker, Nathan, 2-528

Tuke, William, 1-3, 1-84, 1-87, 1-98, 1-100, 3-741

tumor necrosis factor (TNF), 2-398, 3-646

Turner, W., 2-517

Turner, William, 2-438

two-dimensional electrophoresis, 3-553, 3-554, 3-556, 3-557, 3-559, 3-563, 3-564

tybamate, 2-12

typhoid fever, 2-448

U

Ucha-Udabe, Ronaldo, 1-xxviii, 3-789

ulcerous disease, 3-464–3-466

unconscious self, 1-16

unconsciousness, 2-333, 3-491, 3-608

unipolar depression, *see* major depressive disorder

United States Pharmacopeia, 1-364, 1-365, 2-271, 2-272, 2-461, 2-508

up-regulation, 3-634

ural, 1-139, 1-146

urea, 1-110, 1-119, 1-505, 2-182, 2-183, 2-267–2-269

urethane, 1-139, 1-140, 1-149–1-152, 1-158, 1-220, 1-352

urethra, 1-122

urinary incontinence

stress, 2-176

urogenital abnormalities, 3-131

urticaria, 3-466, 3-467

uterus, 1-14, 1-45, 1-73, 1-122, 1-462, 2-545, 3-332, 3-439, 3-732, 3-762

V

vagina, 1-122, 2-435

Vakil, Jal, 2-29, 2-34

Valenciano, Luis, 3-723
Valentin, Gabriel Gustav, 1-190
valerian, 1-69, 1-104, 1-119, 1-125, 1-129, 1-137, 1-143, 1-150, 1-151, 1-159, 2-361, 2-454, 2-455
    Valeriana officinalis, 2-361, 2-454, 3-797
Valeriana officinalis, *see* valerian
Valerianaceae, 2-454
Valerianate of ammonia Pierlot, 1-142
valerianic ether of menthol, *see* brom-validol
valeric acid, 1-119
valerophenone oxime, 1-341
Validol, *see* validolum
validolum
    Validol, 1-146, 1-147, 1-150, 1-151
Valium, *see* diazepam
Vallejo-Nágera, Juan Antonio, 3-715, 3-723, 3-731
Valnes, Kølbjørn N., 3-464
valproate, 1-364, **2-189**, 2-190–2-193, 2-197, 2-206, 2-210, 2-211, *see also* valproic acid
    Depakene, 2-192
    Depakine, 2-191
    Depakote, 2-192, 2-313
valproic acid, 1-329, 1-334, 1-379, **2-189**, 2-189–2-193, 2-196, 2-197, 2-203, 2-204, 2-206, 2-208, 2-209, 2-367, 3-513, 3-514, 3-517, 3-518, *see also* valproate
    Convulex, 2-192
    Depakote Sprinkle, 2-192
valpromide, 2-191, 2-192, 2-194
    Depamide, 2-191
valyl, 1-150
van der Kroef, C., 3-64
vanadate, 1-152
vanadium, 1-147
Vandermonde, Jacques François, 1-66

Varenne, Mauduyt de la, 1-74
vascular medicines, 1-130
vasoconstriction, 2-349
vasodilation, 1-346
Vata, *see* Ayurveda
Vavasseur, Pierre, 1-119
Veda, *see* Ayurveda
Vedic, *see* Ayurveda
vein, 1-69, 1-203, 1-408, 1-488, 2-63, 2-64, 2-413, 2-497, 3-511, 3-667
Velázquez, Andrés, 1-46
Velpeau, Alfred, 2-442
venereal disease, 2-516, 2-523, 3-722
venlafaxine, 1-343, 1-352, 1-360, 2-137, 2-168–2-171, 2-174, 2-176, 2-197, 3-315, 3-316, 3-453–3-456, 3-459, 3-460, 3-562, 3-666
    Effexor, 2-169, 2-171
ventral, 1-199, 1-410, 1-528, 1-530, 1-531, 3-401, 3-638
ventricle, 1-48, 1-52
veratrine, 1-130, 1-151
veretrine sulphate, 1-146
Veronal, *see* barbital
vertigo, 1-120, 1-121, 1-127, 1-136, 1-141, 1-145, 1-156, 1-160, 2-173, 2-333, 2-448, 2-511, 3-739, 3-740
Vesalius, Andreas, 1-64, 1-183
Vetalar, *see* ketamine
vigabatrin, 1-329, 2-204, 2-209, 2-311, 2-314
    gamma vinyl-GABA (GVG), 2-311, 2-314
Vilanova, Arnau de, 1-46, 1-52, 2-491, 3-735
viloxazine, 1-341, 1-360
Vin Mariani, *see* wine
vinbarbital, 1-160
vinconate, 3-656
vinocnate
    seealsovincamine, 3-656

viral vector, 3-570
Virchow, Rudolf, 1-188
visceral, 1-249, 3-432, 3-595
Vishnu, *see* Ayurveda
vision, 1-8, 1-11, 1-41, 1-53, 1-87, 1-88,
       1-101, 1-126, 1-161, 2-150,
       2-159, 2-511, 3-121, 3-122,
       3-606, 3-706, 3-709, 3-711,
       3-732
vitamin A, 3-364
vitamin B3, 2-5, 2-311
Vivactil, *see* protriptyline
Vives, Juan Luís, 1-58, 3-708, 3-735
volinanserin
    MDL-100907, 3-652
Volstead Act (1919), 2-356, 2-419, 3-201,
       3-202, 3-208
Volta, Alessandro, 1-74
voltammetry, 1-174, 1-367, 1-368
Voluntal, 1-158
von Apathy, 1-201
Von Economo encephalitis virus, 2-38
Von Euler, Ulf S., 1-154, 1-205, 3-786
von Gerlach, 1-191
von Liebig, Justus, 1-110, 1-118, 2-4, 2-
       253, 2-254, 2-266, 2-363, 2-494
von Meduna's technique, 3-346, 3-347
von Meduna, Ladislas Joseph, 1-xxiv, 2-
       5, 2-276, 2-335–2-337, 3-344,
       3-347

W

Wöhler, Friedrich, 1-110, 2-455
Würzburg, 1-188
Wagner-Jauregg, Julius, 2-70, 2-338, 2-
       339, 2-405–2-407
Wakefield, Jerome C Johannes Wier, 3-
       326
Waldeyer, Heinrich Wilhelm von, 1-198
Walkington, D.L, 2-534
Walpole, Horace, 3-359
Walters, Verónica Larach, 3-801
Wasson, Robert Gordon, 2-466

Waters, Ralph M., 2-279
Watts, James Winston, 2-343
Weber, Ernst Heinrich, 3-436
Weiner, Richard, 3-351
Weiss, Mary, 3-249, 3-250
Weizsäcker, Viktor von, 3-712
Wells, Horace, 1-305, 2-442, 2-443
Wesley, John, 2-334
Westphal, Karl, 1-14
wet, *see* phencyclidine
wheat horn, *see* ergot
white bang, *see* cannabis
white matter, 1-191, 1-192, 1-442, 1-443,
       1-445, 1-451
Wikler, Abram, 2-308
wild rue, *see* harmal
Wilhelm, Max, 2-135
Wilkins, Robert W., 2-29, 2-30
Williams, George C., 3-415
Willis, Thomas, 1-14, 1-65, 1-186
Willner, P., 1-170
Wilson, Edward Osborne, 3-412
wine, 1-xxiii, 1-xxvi, 1-37, 1-42, 1-50, 1-
       51, 1-68, 1-119, 1-135, 1-140,
       2-110, 2-265, 2-348, 2-414,
       2-432, 2-451, 2-452, 2-455,
       2-490–2-492, 2-494–2-498,
       2-515, 2-516, 2-527, 2-528,
       3-185, 3-204, 3-208, 3-436,
       3-437, 3-494, 3-495, 3-735
    Amargós's Vital Wine, 1-145
    Banyuls, 1-140
    Bordeaux, 2-527
    Mariani wine, 2-455, 2-478, 2-527,
       2-528, 3-198
    transporting, 2-492
Wing, John K., 3-323
withdrawal, 1-406, 1-407, 1-422, 1-
       508, 1-530, 2-159, 2-185,
       2-240, 2-274, 2-277, 2-281,
       2-285, 2-295, 2-296, 2-299,
       2-306–2-310, 2-313–2-316,
       2-326, 2-350, 2-363, 2-405,

2-514, 2-519, 2-555, 2-559, 2-560, 3-11, 3-48, 3-58, 3-61, 3-63–3-65, 3-67, 3-68, 3-140, 3-174, 3-186, 3-205, 3-226, 3-246, 3-250, 3-298, 3-385, 3-471, 3-474, 3-662, 3-665, 3-666, 3-772

withdrawal syndrome, 2-306, 2-559–2-561, 3-287, 3-385, 3-492, 3-498, 3-773, *see also* abstinence syndrome

Withering, William, 2-329
Wood, Alexander, 2-509
Woodward, Robert B., 1-154, 2-32, 2-454
Woodward, Samuel B., 2-326
Wordsworth, William, 2-440
World Psychiatric Association (WPA), 1-xxviii, 1-21, 3-79, 3-108–3-110, 3-137, 3-158, 3-256, 3-296, 3-794
wormwood (Artemisia absinthium), 1-42
wounds, 1-44, 1-121, 1-416, 2-62, 2-431, 2-458, 2-499, 2-506, 3-190, 3-217, 3-294
WPA, *see* World Psychiatric Association (WPA)
Wright, Charles Romley Alder, 2-416, 2-475, 2-510, 3-24

X

Xanax, *see* alprazolam
xanomeline, 3-654
xanthene, 1-311
xanthine, 3-796
xanthoxylum, 2-306
Ximovan, *see* zopiclone
XTC, *see* MDMA (methylenedioxymethamphetamine)

Y

yellow melilot, 1-129

yohimbine, 1-462, 1-463, 1-514, 3-667, 3-668
Yonkman, Frederick F., 1-154, 2-32, 2-454

Z

Z-drug, *see* zopiclone
zaclopride, 3-653
zaleplon, 1-324, 2-293, 2-297–2-299, 3-665
  CL 284,846, 2-298
zalospirone, 2-246
zaprinast, 3-635, 3-638
Zarifian, Édouard, 3-154
Zelmid, *see* zimelidine
zimelidine, 2-148, 2-159, 2-160, **3-63**, 3-63, 3-128
Zimovane, *see* zopiclone
zinc flowers, 1-73
ziprasidone, 1-314, 1-358, 2-98, 2-193, 3-506
Zoloft, *see* sertraline
zolpidem, 1-324, 2-239, 2-293, 2-295–2-299, 3-662, 3-663
  CL-218,872, 2-238
zonisamide, 2-210
zopiclone, 1-324, 1-361, **2-293**, 2-293–2-295, 2-298, 2-299, 3-665
  RP-27267, 2-293
Zorrilla, Francisco de Rojas, 2-438
zotepine, 1-321, 2-98, 3-653
zuclopenthixol, 2-87, 2-88

www.ingramcontent.com/pod-product-compliance
Lightning Source LLC
Chambersburg PA
CBHW081508200326
41518CB00015B/2430